Womanwise

Every Woman's Guide to Gynaecology

Peter Saunders MB, BS, MRCOG
Consultant Gynaecologist

Womanwise

Every Woman's Guide to Gynaecology

Pan Original
Pan Books London and Sydney

To my secretary, Lynne Gardner, and Elaine Levine who typed
and retyped much of the manuscript, to my colleagues and
friends who helped enormously with suggestions and criticisms
and to my wife, Stephanie, who painstakingly read and helped
to edit the work, I am sincerely grateful.

Finally I dedicate this book not to a woman but to a man –
my father – who by example has taught me so much.

Peter Saunders
London 1980

First published 1981 by Pan Books Ltd,
Cavaye Place, London SW10 9PG
© Peter Saunders 1981
ISBN 0 330 26374 9

Printed and bound in Great Britain by
Hazell, Watson & Viney Ltd, Aylesbury, Bucks

Contents

the nipple; nipple rash; breast infections;

'The degree of success of treatment in medicine depends as much on education and motivation of the patient as it does on drugs and surgery – Lord Platt, President, Royal Society of Medicine, 1972

Introduction

This book is about the way you are, the way your body works and why. It covers all aspects of the female reproductive organs except the management of pregnancy about which much has been written.

Modern woman is aware and inquiring, she obviously wants to be involved in decisions affecting her health and future, and to understand the principles of medical treatment. Often such decisions are obvious, for example the use of antibiotics for infection, surgical exploration for a pregnancy in the tube, or radium treatment for certain cancers. However, the choice of a suitable contraceptive, the management of an unwanted pregnancy or whether hormone replacement with oestrogen after the menopause is justified, are topics that demand a more subtle approach as there may be several solutions.

Articles in the papers and documentaries on television can be both relevant and absorbing but may cause concern by extolling the virtues and warning of the dangers of similar treatments. Well-meaning friends or relatives often confuse further with personal anecdotes. How often has a woman refused to accept the idea of an intra-uterine contraceptive because her cousin became pregnant, or her sister's coil disappeared? Or dreaded a sterilization procedure because of a fear of loss of femininity or sexual desire? Or worried herself unduly about a cervical smear test that had to be repeated?

The incentive to write this book has come from you – the reader – and my purpose is to provide a simple explanation of the normal workings of the female body; what can go wrong and what can be done to help; and to attempt to remove the mystique and misconceptions about medicine in general and gynaecology in particular.

1 The sexual and reproductive organs

The outer genital organs

Unlike the sexual and reproductive organs of a man those of a woman are almost entirely hidden by the pubic hair which starts on the front of the body near the legs at a soft pad of fatty tissue called the mons, or 'little hill', which overlies the pubic bone. In a woman the pubic hair on the abdomen stops in a straight line, while in a male the hair can stretch up the abdomen to reach the navel. The quantity and texture of the pubic hair varies with each individual and with racial background, those from Mediterranean countries tending to have thicker and coarser body hair than Western women.

Apart from an obvious protective function the pubic hair serves to retain the aroma produced by the small glands in the pubic area during sexual excitement. Hair appears at the time of puberty when the ovaries first become mature and produce their hormone oestrogen. After the menopause, when the ovaries degenerate and the amount of oestrogen decreases, the hair usually becomes thinner and straighter. Another substance which is responsible for the female growth of hair is called testosterone – a male hormone present in very small amounts in all women and coming from a small organ called the adrenal gland that sits above the kidney.

The external female genital organs consist of several structures which surround the entrance to the vagina collectively known as the vulva. The outer lips (labia majora) of the vulva are two folds of skin joined together at the mons. These lips are really a protective cushion for the vital structures, and keep the inner area moist. The size of the lips again varies with age; in the

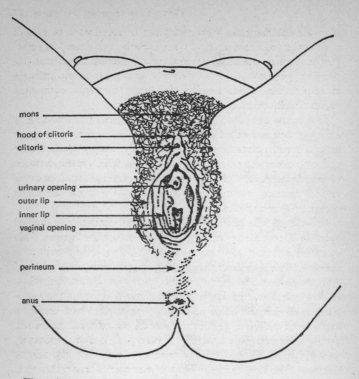

mons
hood of clitoris
clitoris
urinary opening
outer lip
inner lip
vaginal opening
perineum
anus

The vulva

very young and old these lips are small and thin; during sexual reproductive life they are larger and thicker as fatty tissue is present under the skin.

Running along the inner edge of the outer lips are two elongated folds of tissue called the inner lips (labia minora). The inner lips are much thinner and contain no fatty tissue; they fuse together just below the mons but also surround the clitoris to form its foreskin.

The clitoris is a small bud-shaped organ which is the exact equivalent in the female of the male penis and is the most sensitive area of the female body. Although most of the clitoris is usually hidden from view its tip can be recognized as a small pink fleshy projection at the point where the two inner lips meet. Just as the male penis can become erect following sexual stimulation so the clitoris, which is extremely sensitive to touch, enlarges in response to stimulation by the finger or penis, ultimately producing the orgasm.

Just below the clitoris and between the labia minora there is a cleft or opening called the vestibule which contains two openings: a small urinary opening which connects by a short tube to the bladder; and a larger vaginal opening which is the entrance to the vaginal canal. Because the urinary opening is so close to the vaginal opening irritation and infection of the urine can occur occasionally after prolonged or vigorous intercourse.

In women who have not had sexual intercourse the vaginal opening is covered by a thin membrane called the hymen. This membrane is thin and very stretchy and has several very tiny openings through which the blood from menstruation may pass. The shape and size of the hymen varies with each individual and it is usually stretched or torn during a first attempt at intercourse. Often the hymen has already been stretched either by the use of tampons or during certain recreational activities. Young girls who do a lot of horse riding often find it relatively easy to use tampons as the hymen may stretch with this sort of exercise. The tearing of the hymen that occurs during the first act of intercourse usually causes a little discomfort and perhaps some bleeding which usually stops very soon. Even today, women from the Arab world must satisfy their husbands that they come to the marriage bed virginal and the presence of blood after intercourse on the wedding night may still be regarded as proof that the hymen was intact before marriage and previous intercourse has not taken place.

Just inside the vaginal opening on either side are two small bodies or glands called Bartholin's glands which are important because they may occasionally become infected and give rise to a tender swelling which may need surgical treatment (see Chapter 4). The natural function of these glands is to supply lubricating fluid during intercourse.

Finally, there is the external opening called the anus through which faeces pass from the rectum to the outside, and between the anus and the lower part of the vestibule of the vagina is a triangular area of skin covering muscles which are stretched and may be deliberately cut during childbirth in order to make more room for the baby's head to be born. This area is called the perineum.

The internal sex organs

These comprise the vagina, the uterus or womb, the ovaries, and the fallopian tubes or oviducts.

The vagina

The vagina is a passage leading from the vulva upwards towards the uterus. The adult vagina is about 10 to 12 cm long and because it is made up of muscle tissue it is capable of great distension. Normally the walls of the vagina which are lined with folds of skin lie close together. During sexual intercourse the vagina will stretch to accommodate the penis and during childbirth will distend enormously to allow a baby to be born.

During reproductive life the walls of the vagina are usually moist, particularly during sexual arousal, allowing the penis to slide easily into the vagina. The moistness is usually under hormonal influence and is the result of a constant shedding of very tiny cells from the vagina and also a small and constant outpouring of fluid from the neck of the womb at the top of the vagina. This fluid also serves as a protection against infection, lubricating the vagina and keeping it clean. This self-cleansing property makes the formerly popular vaginal douching an un-necessary procedure. In the years before puberty and after the menopause when the hormone influence on the vagina declines the moistness disappears, the walls can become dry and brittle, and the vagina is more prone to infection.

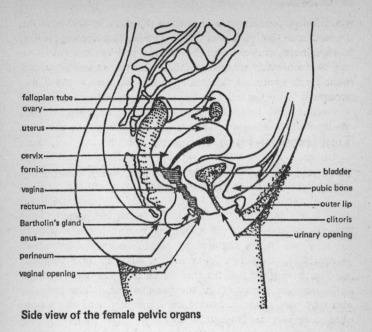

fallopian tube
ovary
uterus
cervix
fornix
vagina
rectum
Bartholin's gland
anus
perineum
vaginal opening

bladder
pubic bone
outer lip
clitoris
urinary opening

Side view of the female pelvic organs

The uterus or womb

The uterus is a hollow muscular organ shaped rather like an upside-down pear, consisting of an upper part, the body, tapering to its lower portion, the cervix or neck. The normal uterus is about 9 cm long and 6 cm across its widest part and weighs about 50 g. During a pregnancy, under the influence of the female hormone oestrogen, the uterus stretches enormously and may come to weigh some thirty times more than the normal.

The cervix projects about 2 cm into the vagina and is thereby readily accessible for examination. It can easily be seen by a torch inserted into the vagina and can be located by the doctor's examining finger, allowing inspection for any abnormalities and also a smear test to be done by gently scraping the surface of the cervix with a wooden spoon so that the cells from the cervix can be examined under a microscope (see Chapter 13). Women can be taught to feel their own cervix by inserting the fingers into the vagina if, for example, they are using a contraceptive cap which needs to fit snugly around the cervix preventing access by the male sperm (see Chapter 8), or need to check the thread of an intra-uterine device. The cervix feels rather like a nose with a small dimple in its centre through which menstrual fluid emerges. This entrance through the cervix into the uterus is usually very small – about the diameter of a fine straw – so there is no danger of a tampon slipping through the cervix into the womb. In pregnancy, however, and particularly during childbirth the cervix is able to expand to such an extent that a baby's head can pass through.

The remainder of the uterus, the body, lies usually bent forward at an angle of 90° to the vagina and is made of thick stretchy muscle on the outside and a hollow cavity which connects with the cervix below and the fallopian tubes on either side at the top. It is along this cavity that the sperm pass in order to gain entrance into the fallopian tube. The cavity is lined by very special cells that are frequently shed and rebuilt during the process of menstruation.

The uterus is kept in its position by a sling of muscle tissue and ligaments spread to the side of the bony pelvis rather like a fan. These supports have great stretch ability allowing the uterus to expand and grow during a pregnancy. With advancing age and after repeated childbirth the supports can lose some of their elasticity and become weak so that the uterus sags, resulting in a dropping or prolapse (see Chapter 7). It is important to realize that the uterus is merely a cradle for the baby and has virtually no hormone function of its own; this is why removal of the uterus or hysterectomy does not cause any alteration in femininity, sexual appetite, or cause hairs to grow on the face and body. The only change that occurs after hysterectomy is that periods no longer exist.

Some women are born with a double uterus due to an error in the way growth occurs in the very early stages in the life of an embryo. The uterus may be split into two in its upper part only or completely separated into two distinct parts with no inter-

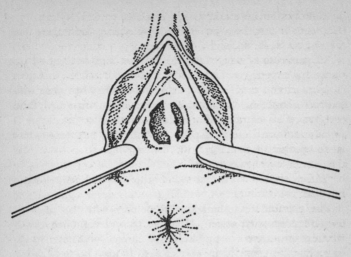

A double vagina

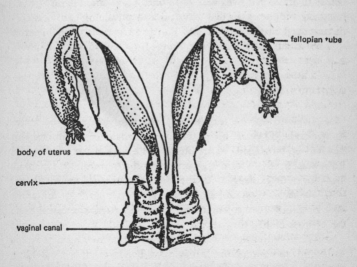

fallopian tube

body of uterus

cervix

vaginal canal

A double uterus

communication. Generally the cervix and vagina are single but occasionally two separate cervices are present and there may also be two separate vaginal entrances.

In such cases, menstruation, ovulation and conception (see later this chapter) occur normally. The abnormalities usually go unnoticed and may cause no complaints. They are most often only diagnosed incidentally on routine examination or in pregnancy. There is a slightly higher risk of miscarriage or premature labour and during later pregnancy the baby may be forced to lie in such a position as to make normal delivery difficult so that Caesarian section may be necessary.

Extremely rarely the uterus and other internal genital organs may be so immature that normal growth is never achieved, or it is also possible for an individual to be born with part male and part female sexual organs. Here the true sex at birth can be accurately determined by blood and chromosome tests so that the child is reared in its correct sex. It may be necessary to remove some of the genital organs of the wrong sex and stimulate those of the correct sex with hormones. Treatment is directed to restoring anatomy so that physical and physiological normality is achieved in the correct sex. Plastic surgery later in life may permit satisfactory sexual intercourse but fertility is not achieved.

The ovaries

The ovaries are the female egg cells equivalent to the testes in the male. They are about the size and shape of an almond and located on either side of the uterus. The ovaries have a two-fold function: firstly to form eggs, and secondly to produce the female sex hormone oestrogen. In the child the ovaries are small and delicate structures, and after puberty they enlarge to the adult size of about 3.5 cm long and 2 cm wide. After the menopause or change of life they shrink to become half the normal adult size. The ovaries are enclosed in a very fine membrane or capsule and sometimes this capsule swells, forming a fluid-filled cavity or cyst. These cysts can enlarge quite considerably and may need surgical removal. It is the oestrogen formed by the ovaries that is responsible for all the feminine attributes of the mature woman, i.e. fullness of the breasts, feminine contour of the hips and normal growth of the sexual organs.

The fallopian tubes

These are two small hollow tubes extending outwards and backwards from the sides of the upper end of the uterus. The outer ends are funnel-shaped and consist of a number of finger-like processes that lie close to and surround the ovary. It is along one of these tubes that the egg which is shed from the ovary passes once it has been sucked up by the tentacle-like end of the tube. In the human, fertilization of the egg by a male seed can only take place in one of the fallopian tubes. Should conception occur, the fertilized egg is helped along the way by very fine hairs inside the lining of the tube which are constantly moving in one direction. The lining of the tube is very fine, about the width of the lead of a pencil, and the cells bordering the lining are extremely delicate. If the tubes are damaged by infection from bacteria that swim through the neck of the womb into the body and thence to the tube the very thin channel can become blocked, preventing the egg from gaining entrance to the tube (see Chapter 5). Sometimes the egg and sperm may meet in the tube, fertilization may occur, but the fertilized egg may not be able to pass back into the womb to grow as an embryo and becomes lodged in the tube to grow there as a tubal or ectopic pregnancy (see Chapter 9). As well as being a pathway for the sperm and egg the lining cells of the tube form nourishing substances which are essential for growth of the fertilized egg during the first few days of its life in the tube.

There is no need for both fallopian tubes to be present for conception to occur. Some women are born with a single tube only or have had one tube surgically removed for infection or tubal pregnancy. Provided the remaining tube is healthy pregnancy can occur as easily with one tube as two.

Puberty and adolescence

Adolescence, from the Latin word *adolescere* which means to grow, is the period of life during which the child becomes an adult. This period varies in duration from one individual to another but is usually taken to extend from the age of ten to about eighteen. Puberty, again from the Latin word *pubertas* which means adulthood, is really the first part of adolescence and it is the time when a young person starts for the first time to be able to have children. This comes about in a girl because the eggs in the ovaries begin to mature and in a boy the testes start producing sperm. Probably the most important physical development of puberty is menstruation, though a number of other very important physical and mental changes also take place around this time.

During childhood the all important pituitary gland in the brain is concerned mostly with physical growth. At puberty all the activities of the gland are increased and it is usually manifested by a sudden spurt in stature just before or after the periods start. Some sexual differentiation does start in childhood; the nipples of the breasts are usually more obvious in the female than the male even by the age of three and the limbs become plump and round at between six and eight. The bones of the pelvis widen between the ages of seven and eleven, and definite signs of puberty are usually present by the age of nine or ten when the breasts develop even more and become enlarged. Hair growth begins, and usually appears first around the vulva. The body contour changes because fat is laid down in the tissues and there is usually some evidence of dark skin pigmentation on the vulva and even round the eyes, mouth and nipples.

The time at which menstrual bleeding first occurs – called the menarche, the onset of menstruation – varies with different cultures and civilizations. In the Western world puberty has been starting earlier and earlier, but there is still a very wide variety of ages at onset and the first period may occur at any time between the ages of ten and sixteen. The average age in Britain is now twelve and among the factors contributing to an earlier puberty are better living conditions, nutrition and an improved standard of general health which is borne out by the fact that menstruation tends to occur earlier in the higher social classes and in urban surroundings. As well as the physical developments that take place around puberty there are great emotional and psychological changes as childish innocence becomes replaced by self-consciousness and modesty. For the first time the girl is beginning to grow up; she becomes interested in her own appearance; she may be aggressive and rebellious as she becomes imaginative and curious. She finds it more difficult to obey orders and may challenge the authority of parents and teachers. She is looking for independence and perhaps for the first time she will start confiding in others than her mother. She is often embarrassed by a lankiness and awkward movements that occur as growth rate spurts. She may get pimples and blackheads and put on quite a lot of weight. She becomes for the first time aware of her sex, and her impulses are often homo-sexual, manifesting themselves by passions for an older girl or woman and gradually being replaced by interest in the opposite sex.

Delayed puberty

It is important to emphasize that although the average age of puberty in this country is twelve the general changes in the appearance of the girl and the onset of menstruation may be delayed until sixteen or even later and this should give no cause for concern. If, however, menstrual bleeding has not started by the age of sixteen, and especially if there is no obvious breast or hair growth, then the doctor should be consulted. Very rarely puberty fails to occur because of a hormone imbalance, but this is very much the exception (see also Chapter 2).

Precocious puberty

This term is arbitrarily defined as the onset of menstruation accompanied also by the other changes of puberty, such as development of the breasts and hair, before the age of ten. In the great majority of instances this is merely an individual character-istic and there is no particular abnormality. What happens is that the pituitary gland in the brain, which is the conductor of the hormone orchestra in the body, merely matures earlier than usual. If a child has any bleeding from the vagina before the age of ten a visit to the doctor is advisable as although there is usually a simple explanation and no abnormality is found occasionally the doctor will want to perform certain tests to make sure that the hormone system in the body is normal.

Menstruation and ovulation

During the reproductive stage of a woman's life from puberty until the menopause two complicated but precisely timed events occur at regular monthly intervals. The first is ovulation or release of an egg by the ovary; and the second involves the changes in the tissue lining of the womb as a result of that ovula-tion. When a girl is born each ovary already contains 30 to 40 thousand immature egg cells called follicles. Of these not more than 400 to 500 are destined to develop into mature eggs. All the other follicles never manage to ripen properly and shrink to a minute size, becoming lodged in the ovary itself.

All the secondary sexual characteristics which appear around puberty, such as breast growth, hair over the pubis, and fat deposition which start the changes in shape to that of a woman, are under the control of the pituitary gland, and around the age of puberty it is this gland that is also responsible for sending a chemical messenger or hormone to the ovary which is responsible for maturing the egg follicles into their adult form. This hormone is called follicle-stimulating hormone. Once mature, this follicle itself puts out another chemical messenger from the ovary called oestrogen. The very first sign of oestrogen being present shows itself in the development of breast buds, soon followed by other signs of puberty.

Each month during the reproductive years one follicle matures and as it grows it moves towards the surface of the ovary. Under the influence of a second hormone coming from the brain called luteinizing hormone one of the egg follicles bursts and expels its egg. This process is called ovulation and usually occurs around the fourteenth day before the onset of menstruation. Once released the egg is attracted to the tentacles of the fallopian tube by a remarkable chemical attraction and the egg travels down the tube and waits there for the sperm to fertilize it. Although ovulation takes place roughly midway between the periods the precise timing varies in any individual; thus some women ovulate around day 9 or 10 of the menstrual cycle and others as late as day 20 or 21. Because fertilization of the egg can only occur within thirty-six hours of ovulation it is important both for those who wish to conceive and those who are using the temperature method of contraception (see Chapter 11) to have precise knowledge of when ovulation occurs.

Ovulation can often be recognized as a crampy pain on one or other side of the lower abdomen occasionally accompanied by a discharge from the vagina which may be blood-stained, occurring roughly midway between the periods. Many women have no outward sign of ovulation and if it becomes important to locate

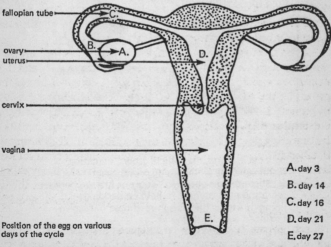

fallopian tube

ovary
uterus

cervix

vagina

A. day 3
B. day 14
C. day 16
D. day 21
E. day 27

Position of the egg on various
days of the cycle

Journey of the egg during the menstrual cycle

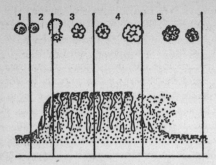

Diagram to correlate the changes in the ovary and uterus during the menstrual cycle and early pregnancy

1. unripe follicle leaves ovary;
   new lining forms in uterus
2. follicle becomes mature;
   lining of womb grows
3. follicle of ovary ruptures (ovulation) (day 12-14)
4. formation of corpus luteum
5. no fertilization occurs — the corpus luteum degenerates;
   the lining of the uterus breaks down as menstrual fluid (period) (day 28)

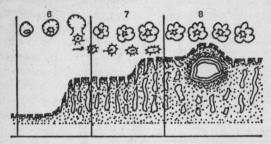

6. new cycle starts, the follicle grows, ovulation occurs and the womb lining grows again
7. fertilization has occurred — corpus luteum persists secreting progesterone to help embedding;
   lining of uterus thickens in readiness to receive fertilized egg (day 14)
8. fertilized egg sinks into the lining of uterus which is thick and spongy;
   menstruation does not occur (day 28)

ovulation certain tests have to be carried out (see Chapter 11).

Ovulation may occur infrequently or perhaps not at all. In the first year or two after menstrual bleeding has commenced it is common for ovulation to occur infrequently until the hormone process of the body has matured sufficiently. This is why periods take a few months to settle into a regular rhythm at first and why true fertility is not achieved at the start of puberty. Because ovulation is infrequent in early reproductive life, the first few periods are usually quite pain-free. Similarly, older women beginning the menopausal years tend to get irregular periods as ovulation becomes infrequent with declining fertility. The causes of failure to ovulate and the management of the condition are fully discussed in Chapter 11.

Once the egg has been released the remainder of the ruptured follicle collapses and changes into a small yellow body called a corpus luteum; it now acquires a new function, producing a second hormone called progesterone, which has an extremely important property involving the preparation of the lining of the womb for the fertilized egg should pregnancy occur. Progesterone prepares the lining of the womb and makes it juicy so that the fertilized egg may be fed and implanted in its lining. Regardless of whether a pregnancy occurs in any particular cycle, progesterone is always secreted after ovulation occurs, causing the womb lining to change in preparation for the fertilized egg. Examination of the lining of the womb is therefore a simple and convenient way of detecting whether the woman is ovulating. Progesterone also raises the body temperature very slightly so that if ovulation has occurred and progesterone has been produced by the fading follicle then the temperature will remain slightly elevated in the latter fourteen days of the menstrual cycle and this is the basis of the temperature test for ovulation (see Chapter 11).

Just as the presence of both fallopian tubes is not vital so one ovary works just as well as two. Ovulation usually occurs from alternate ovaries each month but there is no absolute pattern. If one ovary is removed the remaining organ takes over completely and ovulation should occur every month from the same side with no reduction in potential fertility.

We have seen how under the influence of the follicle-stimulating hormone from the brain the ovarian follicle grows and the ovary produces the female hormone oestrogen. Apart from producing the egg oestrogen also affects the lining of the womb, causing it to thicken and proliferate, and this change occurs on a monthly basis before ovulation, that is to say for the first twelve to fourteen days of the menstrual cycle. After ovulation the hormone progesterone is produced and this causes the lining of the womb to change in consistence as nourishing substances necessary for the implantation of the fertilized egg are produced.

If conception does not occur these hormones – oestrogen and progesterone – gradually dwindle away, the lining of the uterus stops becoming thick and receptive for the fertilized egg, its cells start to shrink and shrivel and gradually disintegrate causing a discharge of blood known as menstruation or the period. Once the period is over the whole cycle is repeated and a new follicle starts growing, forming its own oestrogen, and the lining of the womb again becomes thick and receptive. On the other hand, if fertilization does occur then the two hormones oestrogen and progesterone continue to be put out in large amounts, aiding growth of the fertilized egg and its embedding in the womb. The ovaries then stop forming new follicles and produce less oestrogen and progesterone, a function taken over after the twelfth week by the placenta or afterbirth.

Menstruation continues until the age of forty to fifty when the ovaries gradually shrink with age and become ineffective at liberating the oestrogen; the result is that the periods will cease and this is called the menopause. For a fuller description of the menopause see Chapter 12.

The length of a menstrual cycle, from the first day of one period till the first day of the next, varies between 20 and 36 days, the average being 28; hence the word menstruation derived from the Latin *menses* meaning a month. There is also considerable variation in the duration of bleeding which can last from between two and eight days, four to six days being the average. Once a regular pattern is established each month the time interval between periods is unimportant. Thus a twenty-one-day cycle is just as normal as thirty-five days or twenty-eight days. If, however, the pattern becomes irregular, or if the interval between periods is shorter than twenty-one days or longer than thirty-five, the doctor should be consulted. The most probable explanation is a minor hormone imbalance which often requires no active treatment.

Again, the amount of blood lost during menstruation varies enormously. At an average four to six tablespoons of blood, equivalent to roughly half a teacup, is lost per period. The amount of blood lost will depend on the thickness of the lining of the womb to be shed; for example a girl on the Pill usually has very scanty periods because the Pill prevents ovulation from occurring and consequently the lining of the womb never becomes thick and juicy but always remains rather thin. The menstrual flow consists of a mixture of blood coming from the shed lining of the womb, degenerated cells and a sticky fluid that is an outpouring from the cervix. Menstrual fluid has a particular odour which is not due to the blood itself but is formed by the action of small bacteria that live in the vagina when the blood trickles to the outside. Though it may pass unnoticed it is important to reassure the young girl who starts to menstruate that any aroma is absolutely normal and has nothing to do with hygiene.

Most women experience at least some discomfort during menstruation and in some the pain can be quite severe (see Chapter 2). No one really knows why menstruation can cause discomfort though there are many theories. It has been suggested that the pain is really a spasm or cramp of the womb which contracts during a period under the influence of certain chemical messages or hormones. It used to be thought that pain was worse in girls whose external opening to the cervix was particularly tight. This theory was based on the fact that the pain was often cured once the cervix had been stretched in childbirth, and led to the principle of stretching the cervix under anaesthetic in young girls with severe menstrual pains, thus disrupting the nervous impulses arising from the cervix. This treatment has now largely been replaced by medication (see Chapter 2). Probably menstrual cramp is a result of a number of factors under hormone control and its severity influenced by emotional factors and cultural attitudes.

The most common method for absorbing menstrual fluid is

either with sanitary towels or internal tampons that are introduced into the vagina. Sanitary towels are commonly used in the early years of puberty but by the age of sixteen or seventeen most girls can be taught how to introduce an internal tampon without discomfort. It is not necessary to have had intercourse prior to using the tampon, as the small opening in the hymen that is usually present is large enough to accommodate a small-sized tampon.

Myths and taboos surrounding menstruation are legion and throughout history society has surrounded the menstrual process with mystique and ritual. In primitive cultures menstruation was regarded as evil and dangerous and even today in some parts of the world it is believed that a menstruating woman could damage crops, turn milk sour and even cause animals to abort! For this reason it was common for the woman to be completely isolated from the rest of the community during a menstrual period. There is, of course, no basis for any of these assumptions and it is perfectly safe for the woman who is menstruating to take part in any activity she likes. She can lead an absolutely normal life, including recreational activities, sports, bathing and swimming and sexual intercourse.

Fertilization and conception

Fertilization is the process of fusion of a male seed or spermatozoa with a female egg or ovum. In the human, fertilization must take place in one or other fallopian tube. The ovum which has been shed from the ovary at mid-cycle is attracted to the tentacles at the outer end of the tube by certain chemical substances, enters the lining of the tube and is transported along the tube, partly by the wafting action of minute hairs, and partly by rhythmical contraction of the tube itself. During intercourse about 100 million sperm are ejaculated into the female vagina to start the hazardous journey through the neck of the womb into the cavity and then along the fallopian tube towards the egg. Each sperm, which is about 0.05 mm long, consists of a head and a tail and propels itself quite fast, possibly covering

2.5 cm every eight minutes. Many millions of sperm die on the way and only a few hundred actually manage to find their way into the tube. The remainder disintegrate and die without any harm to the woman.

Only one single sperm is capable of burrowing its way through the shell of the egg. As soon as this happens the head of the sperm separates from the tail and fertilization has occurred. The fertilized egg now forms a barrier which prevents any further sperm from gaining entrance.

Very soon after fertilization the egg begins to divide, first into two, then four and so on, forming a clump of cells called a morula or mulberry which begins to move slowly from the fallopian tube into the uterus where it will grow to form an embryo. Animal experiments suggest that the time taken for the fertilized egg to reach the uterus is between three and five days. Occasionally the fertilized egg is unable to pass back into the uterus and will grow in the fallopian tube to form an ectopic pregnancy (see Chapter 9).

Multiple pregnancies

Multiple pregnancies resulting in twins or triplets are the result of fertilization of more than one egg shed from the ovary. In this country twins occur about once in every ninety pregnancies and tend to run in families, though often missing a generation. Sometimes the egg splits soon after it is fertilized, in which case the twins will be identical, sharing the same sex, features, hair, etc. Non-identical twins are the result of two eggs being fertilized by two sperm, and therefore are unlikely to have the same sex or blood group, and will have dissimilar appearances.

Triplets, quads and quins usually develop from several eggs and therefore tend to be non-identical. Occasionally triplets may be the product of one egg plus one that has split, in which case two of the three may be identical. It is extremely rare for more than three babies to be produced from one act of fertilization. Some fertility drugs given to women who do not ovulate may overstimulate growth from the egg follicle and cause the release of four, five or six eggs which could be fertilized. Because over-stimulation usually only occurs with the complicated, stronger fertility drugs, treatment is usually undertaken in specialized centres where facilities for sophisticated monitoring exist. The closer the control of each woman's response during treatment the less likely she is to produce more than one egg. The commonest type of fertility drug called Clomiphene or Clomid (see Chapter 11) does not produce nearly as strong a response from the ovary and therefore multiple pregnancies are uncommon and rigorous supervision of treatment is usually unncessary.

Boy or girl ?

The human body is made up of millions of cells which develop from a single fertilized egg by a process of dividing many times. As the cells grow they undergo a complicated changing process, from which the different tissues in the body arise. Contained in the centre of each cell is a series of very fine strands called chromosomes, which are responsible for the transmission of all the inheritable qualities of the individual. All the cells of the human body, apart from the reproductive cells, the ovum and the sperm, contain forty-six chromosomes. The reproductive cells differ from the ordinary body cells in that they each contain only twenty-three chromosomes. Twenty-two out of the twenty-three chromosomes are responsible for all the physical characteristics and body functions whereas the remaining chromosome determines the sex. The two sex chromosomes are known as X and Y, because when seen through a very powerful microscope they resemble these letters.

When fertilization occurs the ovary and its twenty-three chromosomes unite with the twenty-three of the sperm, so that a total of forty-six chromosomes is re-established like every other cell in the body. In this way the male and female cell each contribute half of the total, which is why some inherited qualities and characteristics are derived from the father and some from the mother. The sex of the embryo will depend on whether an X or Y chromosome is present in the spermatozoa. Each cell that makes up a woman's body has forty-four ordinary chromosomes and two X chromosomes, whereas a man's body cells have forty-four, an X and a Y. It is the Y cell that is characteristic of a man. If a sperm carrying the Y chromosome fertilizes the egg the new baby will be a boy. If the sperm which fertilizes the egg has an X chromosome the new baby will be a girl. Thus it is the father who determines the sex of the child.

The arrangement of the chromosomes can be detected in any individual by a blood test. The sex of an unborn child can be diagnosed from the fourth month of pregnancy by withdrawing a sample of fluid from the sac enclosing the baby and growing the chromosomes by a special culture technique, amniocentesis (see Chapter 9). Although sex determination by this method is not carried out routinely it may be indicated if one or other parent is a carrier of a congenital disease that affects the male or the female only. In some of these conditions, particularly those involving severe mental and physical handicaps, determining the sex of an unborn child in early pregnancy may be justifiable if termination of the pregnancy is being considered.

Almost certainly the time will come when choosing the sex of the baby will be possible. It is already known that the Y chromosome-carrying sperm which will produce a boy has certain different characteristics from the X which will produce a girl, and experiments have been carried out involving the separation of the male and female chromosome-carrying sperm. It should then be possible to store the sperm by freezing and subsequently to inject the required sexed sperm into the vagina, though as yet this theoretical concept has not proved successful.

Over the years a host of other theories have been suggested for the predetermination of sex of the unborn child. These include altering the acidity of the vagina by douching prior to intercourse, timing sexual intercourse so that fertilization takes place immediately before or after ovulation, having intercourse at certain times of the day or even performing on the top of a mountain or in an aeroplane! There seems little scientific evidence that the timing, frequency, position or location of intercourse has any bearing on the sex of the child.

Points to note

1 The first outward sign of puberty is breast growth which often occurs as early as 9 or 10.

2 The average age for periods to start in this country is 12 but may be delayed until as late as 16.

3 The time interval between periods generally varies between 21 and 35 days with an average of 28. Providing your periods occur with some sort of recurring pattern the interval between them is not important.

4 In most women ovulation occurs 12 to 14 days before their next period whatever the interval between them. In order to achieve a pregnancy intercourse should occur as near to ovulation as possible.

5 There is usually a delay between the start of your periods and the time when you can get pregnant because ovulation does not occur regularly for the first few months of menstruation, *but* it is possible to conceive after the very first period.

6 There is no need to limit any activity, including sexual intercourse, during a period.

7 Fertilization of the egg by a sperm takes place in one or other fallopian tube.

8 Twins are the result of fertilization of one egg which splits into two in which case the twins will be identical, or two eggs fertilized by two sperm producing twins that are dissimilar.

9 There is no foolproof method of ensuring a baby will be born male or female.

2 Problems with periods

Because of the complicated control of menstruation previously described and the many factors involved in ensuring a normal regular menstrual pattern, at certain times in a woman's life the menstrual pattern may change quite dramatically. Usually one of two things happens: either the periods become scanty and irregular or even cease altogether, or they become heavy, recurring at regular or irregular intervals. These changes are particularly common at the extremes of reproductive life, in other words during the first few years of menstruation in the early teens and after the age of forty as the menopause approaches.

Absence of periods (amenorrhoea)

There are three times in a woman's life when periods do not normally occur:

1 Before puberty
2 During pregnancy and after childbirth if breast feeding occurs
3 After the menopause or change of life

The events leading to normal periods occurring in a young girl are usually completed between the ages of twelve to fourteen. Before this time the genital organs are immature or underdeveloped and the chemical messages or hormones necessary to initiate menstruation are not yet produced.

The commonest cause of absence of periods is pregnancy. Here the periods stop because of a rather complicated feed-back mechanism whereby massive amounts of the female hormone oestrogen put out by the ovaries dampen down the production of hormone by the brain which is normally necessary for menstruation to occur. For similar reasons periods may not recommence for some months after delivery of the baby if the mother is breast feeding.

The third time when menstruation may be expected to cease is after the menopause or change of life. This occurs because the ovaries gradually shrink in size and became less and less effective at producing the female hormone oestrogen until eventually all production of oestrogen ceases, causing the periods to stop finally.

Sometimes, however, periods may be absent or may cease at any time due to *abnormal* circumstances. In order to understand why this may occur remember that in the previous chapter it was shown that normal menstruation depends upon a complicated system of messages relayed between the brain, the ovary and the uterus. This pathway is very sensitive, with the result that if there is any abnormality of these organs the uterus may be affected and the periods may not arrive. Let's now look in more detail at some causes of cessation of menstruation.

Some women may be born with certain abnormalities in the chromosome or make-up cells of the body. These congenital abnormalities are not common but they are suspected if a girl is of particularly short stature, perhaps with very scanty or absent hair growth under the arms and in the genital region, and there is often failure of the breast tissue to develop normally. Sometimes the external genital organs are small and remain underdeveloped. There may also be minor abnormalities of the fingers, toes or bones. None of these conditions are harmful but the prognosis from the point of view of fertility and child bearing is gloomy. Some may be diagnosed at birth or soon afterwards if the doctor notices that the baby is born with both male and female characteristics. More usually, however, the problem presents in the early teens when an anxious mother will bring her child along complaining that she has never had a period at all.

A much more common problem is the girl who has menstruated normally but whose periods stop after a variable time for no apparent reason. Why does this happen? Obviously surgical removal or disease of the womb will result in the absence of periods, and in the days when tuberculosis was common the womb and the fallopian tubes were often affected, preventing menstruation. Sometimes the ovaries are very underdeveloped so they cannot produce the sex hormone oestrogen necessary for menstruation. The ovaries may grow and form cysts or innocent enlargements and these alter the sensitive hormone balance of the body. The cysts may give rise to occasional pain or can be an incidental finding by the doctor.

One of the more important causes of failure to have a period is outside influence, such as emotional disturbance at home, embarking on a new career, living for some time in a different country, the death of a close friend or relative, or excessive and rapid weight loss produced by a crash diet. Very rarely small tumours of the brain can cause cessation of menstruation. These are normally found on routine examination on an X-ray of the skull and this is why this investigation is usually requested by the doctor. These tumours are usually innocent and treatable.

Certain medication can cause periods to stop. For instance tablets used for lowering the blood pressure and some used for sedation are known to produce this effect. However, this is almost always temporary and the periods return after treatment has stopped. One of the more important complications of the contraceptive Pill is cessation of periods once the Pill is discontinued. Although this is an all too common finding these days, again it is usually self-righting and the periods return spontaneously after a certain time once the Pill is discontinued. If periods do not recur menstruation may have to be stimulated artificially (see Chapter 11).

Finally, there is an important condition causing *false* absence of menstruation. In other words the girl gets normal feelings that a period is about to start but there is no escape of blood to the outside from the uterus. This occurs because there is some blockage to the menstrual fluid, either at the neck of the womb or sometimes in the vaginal passage and the blood instead of coming out of the vagina actually collects inside the uterus. Every month the uterus will enlarge a little more causing abdominal pain until the girl may complain that she has a tender swelling in the abdomen. The usual cause for this is an imperforate hymen, in other words the hymen or band of tissue closing off the vagina in the young girl has remained intact and does not allow menstrual fluid to pass through. The treatment of this condition involves admission to hospital, examination under anaesthetic and a small surgical incision made into the hymen with immediate escape of menstrual fluid and no resultant disability.

What tests may be done

The first job of the doctor is to exclude the *normal* causes of failure of menstruation: in other words he will need to know whether puberty has not yet occurred, whether the woman is pregnant, or has reached the menopause.

Remember that periods normally start within the pretty wide age range of between ten and sixteen years and almost always before the periods start the breasts grow and sexual hair growth occurs as well. There is great variation in the ages at which these signs, called secondary sexual characteristics, appear and a great variation in the interval between their appearance and the onset of menstruation. This fact is emphasized because so many girls consult their doctors because periods have not commenced when there is no fault present at all. If menstruation has not occurred by the age of sixteen there is no cause for alarm as this may be purely 'delayed menstruation'. After sixteen the girl should see her doctor who will decide whether further investigation is needed and a gynaecological opinion necessary. If breast growth has not occurred by the age of fourteen, or if there is very scanty pubic hair in a girl of particularly short stature, an early visit to the doctor is indicated. Sometimes further investigations are required to find out why the periods are not occurring and usually these take the form of simple swab and smear tests, blood tests and sometimes a 24-hour urine specimen. A chest X-ray and skull X-ray are usual and sometimes admission to hospital may be indicated for a few days so that a full examination may be performed under general anaesthesia together with a scraping of the womb to examine the lining under a microscope. It may be necessary to look inside the abdomen and check the ovaries and internal genital organs; this is done again with the patient fully asleep by inserting a torch called a laparoscope through the navel (see Chapter 14).

If menstruation has started normally but suddenly stops after a variable time, the investigations outlined are usually deferred for a year or so, as periods often come back quite spontaneously during this time. If, however, there is anxiety about child bearing, tests will be done earlier so that treatment can be started.

What treatment can be given

Treatment will depend entirely on the cause of absence of menstruation. Happily the rarer causes, such as chromosome abnormalities for which little can be done, are the exception rather than the rule. Most women whose periods have stopped suddenly without reason can be reassured that no harm at all will come to them and that menstruation will probably recur quite spontaneously after a certain time. If it does become necessary to produce a period artificially so that the egg is released from the ovary this can be done with certain drugs which act by stimulating the rather sluggish brain into putting out the hormone which makes the ovary produce the egg.

Just as periods may suddenly stop altogether for no apparent reason so they may become very scanty with perhaps only a day or two of loss occurring at very infrequent intervals. The problems associated with this condition are really the same as absence of menstruation and similar investigations are required.

Heavy periods

Periods may be heavy in a number of ways. They may come too frequently but are otherwise normal, in other words they last for 5 days every 18 days instead of the usual 28; they may come every month but are very heavy or prolonged and sometimes last for up to 10 days; or they may be heavy and irregular, perhaps coming every 21 days one cycle and 48 days the next. If the main complaint is of heavy periods then the important factor is whether they are coming at *regular* intervals or with no pattern at all, because if they are regular this is usually due to an easily correctable cause, whereas if they are haphazard this may be the first symptom of more serious disease occurring in the womb.

Because patterns of bleeding vary considerably among women it is also important to know whether the excessive bleeding has always been present or whether it is a relatively new complaint. It is therefore helpful to know what quantity of sanitary towels or tampons are used during the period and whether this pattern has suddenly changed. Women often worry about the passage of large clots which look like pieces of liver. This simply means that the bleeding is heavy and it is one of the ways that doctors have of confirming that there has been considerable alteration in the amount of menstrual loss. There is no other significance whatsoever in the passage of these clots.

There are two main reasons why periods become heavy. Either there is a change in the hormone control of menstruation or there may be some physical change in the womb or the ovaries such as fibroids (see Chapter 4), infection (see Chapter 5), or endometriosis (see Chapter 4). An IUD contraceptive may cause the periods to become heavier than usual especially if the woman already has a tendency to have a heavy menstrual loss (see Chapter 8). Hormonal causes of heavy bleeding are due to the fact that the hormones produced from the ovary come out in spurts rather than in a regular rhythm. Because this normally happens at the beginning and end of reproductive life it is quite common to see heavy bleeding at these times. With regard to heavy irregular periods, again the cause may be either hormonal, due to an upset in the production of hormones, or some disease in the pelvis. However, unlike heavy *regular* bleeding which is hardly ever associated with malignancy, *irregular* bleeding may be the first symptom of a little polyp in the womb or even an early cancer. If bleeding, therefore, becomes heavy and irregular this symptom should be reported to the doctor soon.

Treatment

If the periods are heavy but come at absolutely regular intervals there is no need to seek advice immediately, although if the symptoms persist for over three or four cycles then the doctor should be consulted. If the doctor considers that there is no obvious cause in the pelvic organs then a diagnosis of hormone imbalance is usual and this does not always need correcting. If the duration of the period and heaviness start to interfere with normal life, then in the woman under thirty-five treatment usually consists of using one of the contraceptive Pills which take over the menstrual cycle and bring back a normal rhythm. The duration and length of the period is also shortened. If the contraceptive Pill is not suitable the doctor may prescribe pro-gesterone alone which is the hormone that the ovary puts out in the second half of the menstrual cycle and is taken for ten days every month. After three to four months of treatment re-assessment is made and if the desired effect has not been pro-duced then referral to a gynaecologist may be necessary. Some-times admission to hospital is advised in order for a womb scrape (D & C) to be done. This is a minor surgical procedure which enables a scraping from the inner lining of the womb to be taken to ensure there is no obvious cause for the problem inside the womb (see Chapter 14). As well as giving a clue to any disease in the womb the scraping may actually cure heavy periods and, surprisingly, after this minor procedure periods may well return to normal. Heavy periods due to physical causes usually respond to removing the cause, such as removal of an IUD, treatment of infection, etc.

If symptoms persist despite medical treatment and if the blood loss becomes so heavy that replacement with iron tablets is necessary then providing child-bearing years are over the gynaecologist may suggest removal of the womb (hysterectomy).

Irregular vaginal bleeding

So far in this chapter discussion has centred around abnormali-ties of the menstrual period. Sometimes bleeding may occur at any time unrelated to the periods. If bleeding occurs exactly mid-way between the periods this is usually due to shedding of the egg (ovulation) and can be regarded as absolutely normal. If bleeding occurs just before or just after a period this is usually due to a minor hormone change and usually no treatment is required unless it becomes really troublesome. However, if bleeding occurs without any pattern advice should be sought, because this may be the first sign of a small tumour or polyp in the neck of the womb or inside the body of the womb. Both the common forms of contraception, the Pill or the intra-uterine device, may cause some irregular spotting or bleeding which usually settles down in a few months.

Sometimes bleeding occurs immediately after sexual intercourse. In the young girl this is almost always due to the neck of the womb being roughened and this is called a cervical erosion, a harmless finding which often occurs for the first time after childbirth. It is normally treated by cleaning the neck of the womb allowing new skin to grow over the roughened area. In women over the age of thirty-five this symptom should always be reported to the doctor early so that examination may be done to exclude the possibility of a small growth which may be quite innocent but should be treated at an early stage.

Finally, bleeding may occur some months or even years after the menopause or change of life. At the menopause the periods either suddenly stop or they may become a bit irregular or scanty with the interval between them prolonged. Bleeding after the menopause is regarded as significant if it occurs six months after the periods have finished. This is called post-menopausal bleeding. There are numerous causes for it, most of which are harmless and easily treatable. Occasionally, however, this may be the first symptom of more serious disease and for this reason women who bleed after the menopause should consult their doctor without delay.

Painful periods

Most women will experience some discomfort either before or during the menstrual flow, which is usually tolerable. In some, however, the periods are extremely painful and interfere with day-to-day activities.

Menstrual pain may be *primary*, in other words, dating from the early years of menstruation; or *secondary*, occurring for the first time after many pain-free years. In the first type, which is the common one, the pain usually starts within a year or two of puberty. It is cramping in character and felt low in the abdomen and occasionally spreading down the thighs and back. It usually starts just before or together with the menstrual flow and often disappears after thirty-six hours. The severity of this pain is influenced by cultural attitudes, particularly those of the child's mother and family. For example, adolescents in primitive races are said to suffer less severe pain than those in more sophisticated Western societies. Within a single community the incidence of painful periods is higher in the higher social class. Emotional elements in menstrual pain can be strong and the mother may be its source. The family doctor is probably in the best position to estimate this influence.

What causes the pain?
It used to be thought that the cervix was too narrow to allow the menstrual period to escape, a theory that would explain why the periods became less painful with age and after childbirth. For this reason a common treatment for painful periods formerly consisted of stretching the cervix under anaesthetic, a procedure rarely done nowadays.

Recent evidence seems to indicate that the pain is caused by muscle cramps of the uterus as it contracts during a period. These cramps or spasms are in fact caused by stimulation by the hormone progesterone which is released by the ovary after ovulation (see Chapter 1). This would explain why the first year or two of menstruation in a young girl are almost always painless as ovulation does not occur regularly at first, and why the basis for the most successful treatment of painful periods is the contraceptive Pill which prevents ovulation occurring and progesterone from being produced. Examination usually reveals little or no fault and treatment in the first instance should be directed towards education in an attempt to understand the normal processes of menstruation and to correct outdated fallacies and taboos.

Painful periods of the primary type are most frequent in girls who follow sedentary occupations, who do not take enough exercise in the open air, and especially those whose upbringing has been such as to encourage them to regard the menstrual periods as a time when it is dangerous to take a bath or to take part in games. There is good reason to believe, especially from the experience of medical officers of girls' schools, that pain with periods can be largely prevented by normal healthy living – plenty of exercise in the open air at all times as well as during the menstrual period. Menstruation should be regarded as a normal function not a time of illness. There is no reason not to take warm baths, to cycle and dance and to join in such games and exercise as tennis, hockey, and gymnastics during the period. It is interesting to note one study whereby the incidence of painful periods in a girls' school was reduced from 46 per cent to 10 per cent by employing such methods, the 10 per cent consisting mostly of those who did not get permission from their parents to take the necessary exercise. For girls employed in sedentary occupations a brisk daily walk is a useful preventive measure.

Simple pain-relieving tablets may be helpful and the emotional content of the disorder must receive attention if it is significant. If this approach does not succeed and if increasingly strong pain-relieving tablets are necessary then consultation with a gynaecologist is desirable.

The most effective treatment for severe menstrual pain is to stop ovulation occurring with the contraceptive Pill. It is quite remarkable what pain relief this simple treatment will bring but if the girl is unhappy about continuing to take it, after six months she may find that her symptoms have settled even after giving it up. Non-hormonal treatment can also be effective and usually consists of tablets which dampen down the muscular spasms of the uterus. Very occasionally this fails to bring relief and then admission to hospital may be necessary so that the neck of the womb may be stretched.

The secondary type of menstrual pain occurs in later life after many years of pain-free menstruation and is characterized by a general aching discomfort in the lower part of the abdomen which occurs usually a week to ten days *before* a period. There may be an associated headache and general feeling of ill health.

The pain is usually relieved by the menstrual flow but may last throughout the bleeding episode. If periods suddenly become painful following many pain-free years then advice should be sought from the doctor as there is often a physical cause, such as fibroids or endometriosis (see Chapter 4), which is detectable by examination, and treatment will consist of managing the cause.

Pre-menstrual tension (PMT)

This condition has recently become the subject of much interest largely because of its seemingly high incidence. Estimates vary but it is believed that more than three-quarters of all women suffer some of the symptoms of pre-menstrual tension. Formerly believed to be 'all in the mind' there is now good scientific evidence to show that there is a physical cause, and from the result of this discovery treatments have been devised that are simple, safe and very successful.

Women suffering from pre-menstrual tension complain of a variety of symptoms at about the same time each month, usually ten days before a period is due to start. Complaints include painful tender breasts, headaches, nausea and a feeling of fullness in the abdomen. Fatigue, anxiety, irritability and sometimes severe depression are not unusual. There may be sleeplessness, difficulty in concentration, mood swings, restlessness and loss of sex drive. Some women say that they become forgetful, and their judgement is impaired with a lowering of efficiency. Once the periods have started, these complaints usually improve and often disappear completely until ten days or so before the next cycle when the whole process is repeated.

Why does PMT occur?

The basic cause is that the hormones controlling the menstrual cycle are slightly out of balance. In Chapter 1 it is shown that for the first fourteen days of a period the hormone oestrogen is secreted by the ovary, and in the second half of the menstrual cycle, progesterone. It is now believed that one of the causes of pre-menstrual complaints is an imbalance of these two hormones so that too much oestrogen and too little progesterone is produced by the ovary in the second half of the cycle. No one really knows why this happens and PMT often occurs for the first time in the thirties and tends to get worse rather than better with age. Some women find that they only start to suffer from complaints after the birth of their first baby as the whole process of childbirth can sometimes cause the ovary to put out its hormones in a somewhat irregular manner. Pre-menstrual tension stops after the menopause because the ovaries no longer function properly when the periods have stopped. It is important to realize that women who have had a hysterectomy prior to the menopause can also suffer from PMT if the ovaries have not been removed at the same time as the uterus, as the remaining ovaries will still work for a number of years and will therefore continue to provide the cyclical hormone changes, though of course there can be no periods.

Hysterectomy, therefore, does not necessarily cure the symptoms of pre-menstrual tension.

What treatments are available?

The type of treatment will depend on the severity of the complaint. Some women with mild symptoms are able to do much to relieve their own symptoms by reducing stress, learning to relax and understanding why pre-menstrual tension occurs. If the symptoms are moderate or severe then the family doctor should be consulted.

There are three treatments that are commonly used. The first treatment consists of taking a course of fluid-removing or diuretic tablets for the ten days leading up to a period, as the hormone imbalance causes surplus fluid to be formed particularly in the legs and breasts. Provided treatment is kept to a relatively short time there are no complications, though if taken over a long period diuretic tablets can cause some disturbance of the water-regulating mechanism in the body which occasionally upsets the way that the kidneys work.

This treatment has largely been replaced by two specialized groups of tablets. The first involves a course of progesterone tablets which are again taken for the 10 days leading up to a period, as one of the causes of PMT is a deficiency in the level of this hormone at a crucial time in the menstrual cycle. There are several types of synthetic progesterone available and they come in the form of tablets which are available on prescription only and therefore have to be prescribed by a doctor. Treatment is usually recommended for between six and nine months but some women find that their symptoms recur once they stop treatment. If this happens there is no reason why treatment should not be continued for longer, but again the doctor will know what is likely to bring the greatest relief. There are no harmful side effects of progesterone treatment though some women occasionally suffer minor menstrual changes as a result. The periods, however, usually remain regular and progesterone has the added advantage of lightening the menstrual flow which is especially helpful for some PMT sufferers whose periods seem to be heavier.

An alternative treatment, some say equally effective, consists of a special vitamin, vitamin B6 called pyridoxine which is available without prescription from the chemist because it is not a drug in the true sense of the word. Treatment again is usually started about ten days before a period and two tablets of vitamin B6 should be taken and continued until three days after the period has started. Some women benefit from two tablets taken daily for ten days and others need more, and although a prescription from the doctor is not needed, it is wise to consult a practitioner so that he may help gauge the correct dosage for each individual. Vitamin B6 is a completely safe drug with no known side effects and does not interact with any other treatment, so treatment need not be stopped if the contraceptive Pill is being used or if antibiotics are being taken for a coincidental infection.

Although some women get almost immediate relief from their symptoms by taking one or other of the treatments outlined, others take a little time to react or find that some of their symptoms persist after others have disappeared. It may take time to establish the treatment that works best for each individual and to get the dosage right, but it seems that over three-quarters of all women that have received treatment appear to be completely cured or have gained considerable relief from the complaints of pre-menstrual tension.

Points to note

1 During the fertile years pregnancy is the commonest cause for your periods to stop suddenly. Periods will not occur before puberty or after the menopause and are unlikely to return after a pregnancy until breast feeding stops.

2 If you miss a period and cannot be pregnant, before seeing your doctor wait for another month at least, to see if your periods return – they normally do. If you think there is the slightest chance of a pregnancy, as suggested by tingling or enlargement of the breasts or feeling sick, then see your doctor soon.

3 Do not be surprised if your periods become very short when you are taking the contraceptive Pill, this is quite normal.

4 It may take a month or two for your periods to return when you come off the Pill. If you are trying to get pregnant and your periods have not returned within three months go and see your doctor, as sometimes special tablets are needed to bring them on again.

5 Remember that anxiety plays an important part in making periods irregular. It is not unusual for you to miss a few periods following some emotional crisis in your life.

6 Before seeing the doctor about your menstrual problem it is useful to record on a chart your particular pattern of bleeding and its heaviness over a three-month period.

7 Heavy *regular* periods hardly ever imply sinister disease. Heavy *irregular* periods or haphazard bleeding between periods and after intercourse should be reported to the doctor – soon.

8 An IUD contraceptive may cause your periods to get heavier initially. This usually settles within a month or two.

9 Similarly, sterilization by the laparoscope method may

cause heavy periods, particularly if the tubes are cauterized (see Chapters 8 and 11). Remember, however, that the increased flow of blood may not really be heavy; it may just appear to be so, particularly if the periods had been very light before sterilization if the Pill was used.

10 The less notice you take of your periods the less discomfort and pain will be a problem. Periods often become less painful after childbirth.

11 If the degree of pain is such that it interferes with your normal activities seek medical advice – there are very efficient cures.

12 Periods that become painful for the first time in later life usually imply a treatable cause in the pelvic organs.

13 Pre-menstrual tension is a common condition which can often be helped. Don't grin and bear it every month if your life is a misery. Your doctor should be able to help.

3 The breasts

The function of the breast is two-fold. Firstly, to nourish and feed the new-born infant and secondly, it has an erotic function for the attraction of the opposite sex, the emphasis of each varying with different cultures.

The breasts undergo enormous changes in a woman's life. The infantile breast consists purely of a nipple which stands out from a surrounding pinkish area called the areola. By the tenth or eleventh year, as puberty approaches, the areola swells and the breast starts to grow under the influence of the sex hormones oestrogen and progesterone. The milk channels develop from the nipple and divide into smaller and smaller branches and at the same time fat is laid down around the milk ducts so that when puberty is reached the breasts are mature, prominent, rounded and firm.

In reproductive life certain changes occur in the breasts with each menstrual cycle. The milk ducts or channels develop further and fluid seeps into the fatty tissue to cause distension of the breasts which can become quite uncomfortable, particularly in the week preceding a period. The breasts can be quite tender and have a lumpy feel which settles once the period is over. This is, in fact, quite a normal occurrence but occasionally the discomfort in the breasts is intense and this can usually be treated satisfactorily (see later this chapter).

In pregnancy the breasts swell, again become tender, and sometimes the areola changes colour from pink to brown in the early months of a first pregnancy, particularly in brunettes. The milk channels and surrounding tissue enlarge considerably and milk production occurs quite early in pregnancy and it is common for a milky-like substance to squeeze out of the breasts throughout pregnancy. Breast feeding will increase the size of the breasts further and they only usually return to normal size some weeks after breast feeding has finished. After the change of life or menopause the breasts start to droop and become less firm as the sex hormones production by the ovary becomes less and less effective.

Variations in size

Large breasts

Breast size tends to increase with age and many women find that their breasts enlarge after thirty-five. Most of the enlargement is due to deposition of fat through obesity, and excessive fluid retention is a contributory factor. Extreme enlargement of the breasts which causes discomfort and embarrassment, particularly if the breasts are droopy as well as large, is best managed by a well-designed and well-fitting brassière. Hormone treatment is only occasionally successful and cosmetic surgery which involves removing some of the pads of fat may be required if the enlargement is gross.

Sometimes one breast is larger than the other giving an unequal appearance to the chest. This has no special underlying significance.

Small breasts

Breasts may appear small because there is too little hormone stimulation or just because the woman is slim. If no breast tissue develops at puberty at all then the girl should consult her doctor. If there is some breast enlargement there is not much that can be done to increase the size. Rubbing hormone cream into the breasts does little good because small breasts are due to lack of fat and hormone creams do nothing to lay more fat down; they merely enlarge the milk channels. Provided the girl has an upright posture and does not stoop, exercises to strengthen the breast muscles are not very helpful. If the girl has a stooping posture then these muscles can be strengthened, which will give the appearance of the breasts being pushed forward. Just as the breasts may be made smaller by cosmetic surgery so they may be increased in size and this is usually done by inserting a special bag filled with fluid or mould between the breasts and the underlying muscles. Careful thought must be given to any form of cosmetic surgery as the results can sometimes be disappointing. Usually cosmetic surgery has to be done privately but occasionally if there is gross enlargement of the breast tissue due to a medical condition cosmetic surgery may be obtained under the National Health Service.

Is a brassière necessary?
The wearing of a bra is peculiar to the civilized Western woman and successive generations of women have been traditionally advised that there is a need for wearing a bra from puberty in order to promote growth of the breast and to prevent sagging, but there is no evidence that the wearing of a bra influences the way the breasts will grow and this importance has been overemphasized. Certainly during pregnancy and breast feeding the wearing of a bra will increase comfort and women with large breasts will also derive help from a well-fitting support.

Provided the adult breast is normal in appearance and growth there is no medical reason for bra support. However, if a woman feels more comfortable in a bra or feels it enhances her attraction she should wear one.

Abnormal nipples

The nipples of some breasts are turned in or inverted and this is usually due to a developmental fault and requires no treatment at all. Breast feeding may be difficult if the nipples are inverted and it is sometimes helpful to wear firm shell supports which withdraw the nipple somewhat during pregnancy. If the nipples

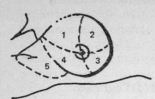

Areas that should be checked

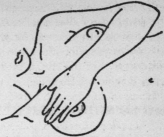

1 Lie on bed, folded towel under right shoulder, right arm behind head. With flat of fingers, feel upper, outer quarter of right breast.

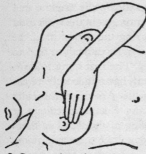

2 Repeat on lower, inner quarter.

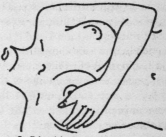

3 Bring right arm to side, and examine lower, outer quarter.

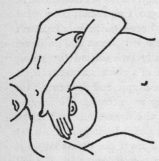

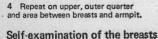

4 Repeat on upper, outer quarter and area between breasts and armpit.

Self-examination of the breasts

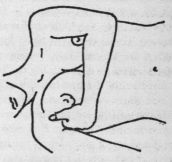

5 Examine armpit.
6 Move towel under left shoulder and repeat the examination on the left breast.

have been normal but one or other starts to invert later in life
then advice of the doctor should be sought. Occasionally extra
nipples occur anywhere along a line from the armpit to the
pelvic bones. Usually they occur in the armpit and no treatment
is necessary.

Self-examination of the breasts

Some lumps in the breast are obvious to see and feel, others may
only be detected on routine examination. Feeling your own
breasts regularly for any swellings is a worthwhile exercise and
easy to do with a little practice. The best time is in the week after
a period because leading up to and during the period itself the
breast will appear lumpy and it is much more difficult to find an
isolated lump or swelling at these times. The first thing to do is
to stand in front of a mirror with the arms hanging loosely by the
sides and look at the outline of the breast. Are the two breasts
similar in size and shape? Is there any change in colour or
appearance of the nipple or any dimpling of the skin? Is there
any discharge or bleeding from the nipple? All these symptoms
may be important.

If the arms are next raised above the head the lower part
of the breast may be seen more easily. Next, the breasts should be
felt for any isolated swellings or lumps. This is best done lying
on a bed or in the bath so that the breast tissue is completely
relaxed. Using the right hand for the left breast and with the
flat of the fingers only, systematically feel around the whole
breast rather as if examining the face of a clock. Concentrate on
the section of the breast between the nipple and the armpit for
this is where cancers most commonly are situated. It is important not to squeeze the breast with the fingers and to use the
flat of the hand because it is easy to feel false lumps which are
in fact parts of the normal breast tissue if the breast tissue is
grasped between the fingers and thumb. Repeat with the left
hand for the right breast.

What to watch for

Pain and swellings in the breast

Earlier in this chapter it was explained that once the menstrual cycles are fully established swelling and a lumpy feeling in the breasts in the week leading up to the period are common. This occurs because of the sex hormones that are liberated around this time and once the period is over the symptoms tend to settle.

As women get older this lumpiness in the breasts may persist and may be a cause of considerable anxiety especially if lumps are noticed in the breasts at other times than during the period. This may send her scurrying off to her doctor because of an overriding fear of cancer. Doctors call this condition of lumpiness in the breasts mastitis and it is usually completely harmless as the lumps that appear in the breasts are hardly ever precancerous especially in child-bearing years. There are two types of mastitis. One form is usually found in the younger age group in the twenties and thirties when there may be mild discomfort and swelling in the breast which is generally worse before a period but remains to a certain degree the whole time. Both breasts are usually involved and when the doctor examines the breasts they have a generalized lumpy feel. A well-fitting bra together with fluid-removing tablets or special hormone tablets to be taken in the week leading up to the period usually gives relief. The other type is often more worrying for the patient because instead of a generalized lumpy feeling in the breasts the woman may detect a single isolated swelling and again her first thought would be 'Have I cancer?' What happens here is that the fluid gets trapped in the milk ducts to form small sacs or cysts which gradually enlarge to form a noticeable swelling. They are often tender to feel and when pinched between the finger usually are quite mobile under the skin. These swellings occur in the later age group and may be found for the first time around the menopause.

Although 75 per cent of isolated swellings in the breast are usually of a completely benign nature this finding should prompt a visit to the doctor especially if they occur in the woman over 40.

Discharge of fluid from the nipple

Throughout pregnancy and for a variable period of time after breast feeding has finished it is quite normal for the breasts to secrete milk, and this may also occur in some women quite unrelated to a recent pregnancy. For example milk production may occur in certain women whose periods stop suddenly due to stimulation of the milk-producing centre in the brain governed by the pituitary gland. Once the periods return, milk ceases to be formed in the breasts.

Rarely, an innocent tumour causes overgrowth of the pituitary gland and subsequent breast activity and milk production. The diagnosis is made by blood tests and X-rays and treatment with a drug (Bromocriptine) that reduces the milk-producing hormone output is generally curative. It is extremely uncommon for surgical removal or irradiation of the tumour to be necessary.

Certain drugs, notably some used for sedation or treatment of allergies, can occasionally cause breast milk production. This is usually an incidental finding, with no special significance, and the milk ceases once treatment is discontinued.

Usually no cause for sudden milk production is found, and though it may last for months or years unless treated, there is no other significance and the breasts stop forming milk spontaneously.

The nipple that has always been turned in or inverted is more prone to be infected, and occasionally swelling, redness and discharge of pus may occur and is treated with antibiotics or by making a small cut into the breast to let the fluid escape. A green or blood-stained discharge from the nipple itself should be taken seriously and be reported to the doctor. Occasionally it is associated with an underlying cancer, not so much of the breast tissue but of the milk channel, and if detected early this form of breast cancer should be curable.

Nipple rash

The skin of the breast is just as liable to become inflamed or prone to eczema as the rest of the body and a rash may occur covering both breasts with irritation causing the woman to scratch. Treatment with special creams is usually curative. If a rash develops in the region of one breast only this may be due to a special skin condition called Paget's disease and a diagnosis has to be made by removing a small piece of skin under local anaesthetic. If Paget's disease is confirmed a further exploration of the breast tissue is undertaken by the surgeon because very occasionally underneath the reddened area there is a very small cancer which usually does not spread beyond the breast tissue itself but nevertheless should be removed.

Breast infections

It is uncommon for infection to occur in the breasts in the course of a pregnancy. Boils or abscesses tend usually to occur in the lying-in period after childbirth and are due to blockage of the milk channels in the breast. Treatment is by antibiotics or drainage of any pus by a small surgical cut.

Cancer of the breast

This will be dealt with in Chapter 13.

Points to note

1 Because the size of your breasts is under the influence of the hormone oestrogen, they will tend to enlarge at times when there is more oestrogen than usual, i.e. during pregnancy and while on the contraceptive Pill, and they may get smaller after the menopause.
2 You should report any sudden change in appearance in one breast or discharge from the nipple.
3 Your breasts often become lumpy and tender in the week before a period and sometimes if you are taking the Pill. If this becomes a real nuisance treatment with progesterone or Vitamin B6 may be helpful.

4 Most swellings in the breast are quite innocent. However, don't ignore a lump that persists after your period. If you are in doubt as to whether a lump exists or not let your doctor have a look.

5 If you think that your breasts are unusually large or small and you are considering advice about cosmetic surgery, make sure you know exactly what the plastic surgeon plans and particularly where any scars will be placed after surgery.

4 Genital swellings

Swellings of the genital organs are common, occur at any age, are usually innocent and may not cause symptoms. Those arising from the external genital organs are usually noticed whereas a swelling of the uterus or ovary may only be discovered on routine examination by the doctor, hence the importance of an annual check, particularly in the later age group.

Not all lumps need treatment but any swelling of the internal or genital area should be reported to the doctor, so that a diagnosis can be made. If a woman notices enlargement of the abdomen or feels a lump in her abdomen an early visit to the doctor is recommended.

Swellings of the outer genital organs

Genital warts

Like warts elsewhere in the body genital warts are caused by a tiny organism called a virus. No one really knows why these warts occur around the vulva and vagina but sexual intercourse seems to be a factor. Formerly called venereal warts because it was thought that they were only transmitted through coitus, warts may occur quite commonly in sexually non-active women and though annoying have no serious consequences. Vaginal warts seem to grow more rapidly in the presence of vaginal secretion and particularly certain types of discharge (trichomonas). They are commoner in pregnancy and in those taking the contraceptive Pill.

At first only one or two warts may be discovered in the skin around the entrance to the vagina and are usually quite tiny. They may grow larger and multiply and sometimes spread into the vaginal canal. Vaginal irritation and bleeding may occur, particularly if warts occur during pregnancy.

Small warts may disappear spontaneously or when an associated vaginal discharge is treated. Specific treatment involves the use of a special paint which causes the warts to shrivel. If this treatment is recommended great care has to be taken to ensure that the paint is not smeared over the skin generally because normal skin reacts strongly to the paint and small burns may occur. Each wart should be painted individually. If this treatment fails to remove the warts they can be completely destroyed by applying a hot loop or wire (cautery) and this is done under a general anaesthetic.

Polyps and cysts

There are many different types of small swellings that appear around the lower genital area arising in the skin or inside the vaginal canal. Some of these swellings contain fluid and are called cysts, and others grow from a stalk and are called polyps; the great majority are completely harmless. Small cysts can grow due to the accumulation of their fluid content and can become infected – causing considerable throbbing pain which will persist until the swelling is opened or removed. A common example is a cyst that appears just inside the vagina on either side distending and distorting the edge of the vulva. Called a *Bartholin's cyst* after the doctor who first described the small gland that lies inside the vagina from which the cyst takes its origin, this swelling can grow rapidly to the size of a golf ball and may become extremely painful if infected. The Bartholin's cyst can disappear if it bursts spontaneously and discharges its fluid, but it will almost certainly recur unless treatment by a surgical incision, involving sewing the cyst wall to the skin, is performed (marsupialization).

Sometimes a polyp can arise from the neck or body of the womb which may grow as the stalk stretches until a swelling appears at the vaginal entrance. These polyps are often symptomless and found by the doctor on routine examination, or they may cause vaginal discharge or irregular bleeding. Usually they are removed under general anaesthetic.

Any swelling that is discovered in the lower genital region should be reported to the doctor. The great majority are totally harmless and reassurance can usually be given that no treatment is necessary or that the lump should be removed. Cancerous swellings in the region of the external genital organs are extremely rare, especially in the woman under fifty-five.

Swellings of the internal genital organs

Fibroids

The wall of the womb consists of muscle tissue which allows it to expand in pregnancy and contract in labour, and fibrous or connective tissue woven closely together giving the womb its strength. Under certain circumstances some of the muscle tissue can form into knots which at first are no bigger than a pea but can grow and multiply, occasionally becoming so large that they cause a swelling which may become obvious to the woman or her doctor during a general examination.

Fibroids are so common that they exist in 25 per cent of all women, although they may not necessarily give rise to problems or even be noticeable. They are much commoner in women who have not conceived or are infertile, a fact that has given rise to the concept that 'fibroids are the rewards of virtue and babies the fruits of sin'! They are also more common in Negroes than in Caucasians. Extremely rare before puberty, fibroids degenerate and get smaller after the menopause, suggesting that their growth may be dependent on the female sex hormone oestrogen. This hypothesis is borne out by the fact that fibroids tend to grow larger when there is a lot of oestrogen in the body, or when contraception is provided by the Pill. Fibroids can be considered to be perfectly benign swellings. Exceedingly rarely can they become cancerous and the diagnosis is usually made in

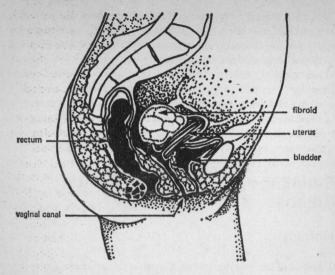

Fibroids in the uterus

retrospect when the pathologist examines the fibroids after they have been removed.

If fibroids do give rise to problems, the commonest complaint concerns the periods which become increasingly heavy. Pain is unusual but large fibroids may press on surrounding structures giving rise to pressure symptoms; for instance on the bladder causing frequent desire to urinate, or on the diaphragm causing heartburn or acid indigestion. Rarely fibroids may grow down into the canal of the womb and be extruded through the cervix, forming a fibroid polyp, which causes irregular vaginal bleeding and sometimes labour-like pains.

Treatment of fibroids

There are three methods of approach. Either no treatment is necessary; the fibroids are removed surgically, leaving the womb intact; or the womb is removed with the fibroids (hysterectomy). Small symptomless fibroids found on routine examination need no specific treatment. Usually reattendance at the local clinic or doctor's surgery is suggested after six months for a further examination to check that no irregular bleeding has occurred and that the fibroids have not grown rapidly. Some surgeons prefer to adopt a more active policy, particularly if no further children are desired, but this is very much a matter of individual choice.

Removal of the fibroids with conservation of the womb is not the usual treatment, for if surgery is required most surgeons will advise removal of the whole womb containing the fibroids. This is because fibroids are very seldom solitary and often there are so many small seedlings embedded in the womb that it is virtually impossible to ensure their complete removal. Removal of the fibroids without sacrificing the womb is normally reserved for the woman who wishes to have further pregnancies and for whom the fibroids have been causing problems with menstruation, or, rarely, when fibroids have been implicated as a cause of recurrent miscarriage (see Chapter 9).

Fibroids and pregnancy

Fibroids that are discovered for the first time in pregnancy usually cause no problems whatsoever to the mother or her baby. They tend to rise out of the pelvis with the womb, though as pregnancy advances the fibroids will inevitably grow and sometimes can be felt quite clearly in the abdomen. They can cause pain for varying spells during pregnancy as they may grow rapidly, and although this is not a serious consequence it is a nuisance. It is unusual for fibroids to cause a miscarriage unless they are sited in the canal of the cervix. However, if two or three consecutive miscarriages occur when fibroids are present, surgical removal in between pregnancies may be justified. The great majority of pregnant women with fibroids are able to have their babies normally. Rarely, fibroids can obstruct the birth canal and cause the baby to lie in an abnormal position. Should this occur the baby may have to be delivered by Caesarian section. After pregnancy the fibroids soon shrink to their original size though they will not necessarily disappear completely. If surgery is indicated for fibroids this is usually deferred for at least three months after the birth of the baby.

Cysts of the ovary

Every month at the time that the egg is shed, the ovaries can become distended and enlarged. Because the lining cells of the ovary form fluid and the whole ovary is contained within a very fine bag or capsule, distension of the ovary can form a cyst. Usually these cysts do not grow large and go unnoticed. Sometimes they enlarge to the size of a hen's egg or larger in which case they may cause pain in the abdomen as the fluid inside the cyst swells, causing distension of the sac surrounding the ovary. This is one of the reasons why discomfort exists in the few days before a period or around the middle of a cycle when ovulation occurs.

Routine examination may reveal an enlargement of one or other ovary, and provided that the cyst is not more than a few centimetres in size no treatment is necessary as it will shrink after the period and any discomfort with pass away. These cysts are not due to any disease process but simply result from an exaggeration of the normal menstrual cycle whereby the hormones responsible for producing the egg make the ovary grow at the same time.

The ovary, however, is a complex structure consisting of many types of different cells, all of which, at any time, can cause enlargement of the ovary and cyst formation. Again, they may go unnoticed or may be found on routine examination by the doctor. If these cysts are small and cause no symptoms no treatment is necessary and reattendance in a few weeks or months will be necessary to ensure that the swelling has not grown in size. Sometimes the ovary can grow, causing a swelling in the abdomen or abdominal pain.

Unlike fibroids which hardly ever become cancerous, cysts on the ovary can slowly develop malignant change which can only be discovered after the swelling has been removed and examined by the pathologist. Largely because of this fact it is common practice for an exploratory operation to be advised for cysts over a certain size that do not disappear.

The surgical procedure will depend on the age of the patient, the appearance of the ovary, the likelihood of an early cancer and whether or not the other ovary is normal. In a young girl with a cyst that appears innocent it is common practice to shell-out the cyst and leave the ovary intact. Sometimes the surgeon will remove the whole ovary including the cyst, and providing the other ovary is normal this will in no way impair the important secretion of the female hormone oestrogen as the single ovary takes over the function of two perfectly.

If a woman over forty who has finished her family is found to have a cyst of the ovary the surgeon may suggest that not only the ovary containing the cyst but the other ovary and possibly even the womb should be removed as well. Although this treatment may sound a bit dramatic it is usually suggested as a preventative measure to exclude the possibility of a further cyst arising on the other ovary or of a possible early malignancy in the ovary that may later involve the womb. The various possibilities will of course be discussed before any surgery is undertaken so that the woman knows what her particular gynaecologist feels and she will be made fully aware of the various alternative surgical procedures.

Endometriosis

This is a strange disorder usually affecting women in the older age group who have not had children. The term endometrium is a word used to describe the inner lining of the womb, and in endometriosis parts of this inner lining form into small clumps which may grow under the influence of the female hormone oestrogen which is continuously being secreted by the ovaries throughout the reproductive years. As these individual lumps grow they tend to fuse so that the whole womb can become enlarged. The trouble is that the condition is not necessarily confined to the womb itself because tiny fragments or nests of this endometrium can get forced back along the fallopian tubes with menstrual blood and drop out of the open end of the tube to lie on neighbouring structures, such as the ovary or sometimes the bladder and the rectum.

Because the endometrium acts as a foreign agent these organs will react in different ways. The ovary will swell and may form cysts, but instead of the cysts containing fluid they will contain altered blood and this will almost certainly give rise to pain, mainly occurring in the week or ten days preceding a period. If little drops of endometrium become scattered over the pelvic tissues, particularly the ligaments or guy-ropes that keep the womb in its normal position, the womb will be pulled downwards into the backward position (see Chapter 7) causing lower abdominal pains and backache, particularly during sexual intercourse. Also the periods will tend to become heavy. The womb, the ovaries and the tubes may all become rather glued together and the tubes may be stuck to the back of the womb so that their ends may be blocked, preventing passage of the fertilized egg and leading to infertility.

Endometriosis may be confined to the womb itself or one or other ovary or may involve all the pelvic tissues, and the diagnosis can only be made for sure by inspecting the abdomen through the laparoscope or a small surgical operation.

A combination of painful periods, usually worst in the week before the flow and often relieved when menstruation starts, periods that have become heavier than usual, nagging backache and pain on deep penetration during sexual intercourse, all occurring for the first time in the infertile woman over thirty-five, might typically be diagnosed as endometriosis.

Treatment of endometriosis

Formerly the only recognized treatment was radical surgery, often resulting in a young woman having to sacrifice her chances of becoming pregnant. Nowadays the condition can largely be arrested by hormones and the contraceptive Pill is quite effective. Other medical treatments include a progesterone hormone alone – the sister drug of oestrogen – given in a dose sufficiently high to stop the periods completely for a few months and this treatment is effective in dampening down deposits of endometriosis. Hormone treatment was first suggested after several researchers noticed an improvement in the symptoms of women suffering from endometriosis during pregnancy, and equated this to the high output of hormones, particularly progesterone, which occurs naturally during pregnancy. Treatment may be discontinued after some months, particularly if fertility is in question, in the hope that conception will occur soon. There are also newer, more specific drugs which act by lowering the natural hormone production of the pituitary gland, and these drugs though expensive have been shown to be particularly effective in controlling pain.

If laparoscopy or inspection of the abdomen via an incision reveals extensive endometriosis involving the ovaries and other tissues of the body, and if symptoms of pain and heavy periods are severe, surgical removal of the affected organ may be indicated. If infertility is not desired, surgery will be kept to a minimum; if child bearing is not a factor, or if the disease has spread to involve all the pelvic organs, then removal of the womb with both ovaries and tubes may be the only solution. Fortunately, with medical treatment becoming increasingly effective this sort of radical surgery is becoming less common and if the ovaries have to be removed the sex hormone oestrogen can be replaced in tablet or implant form (see Chapter 14).

Points to note

1 If you notice a lump in the region of the vulva or you think that your abdomen has enlarged let your doctor have a look. Not every lump needs to be removed but a diagnosis needs to be made.
2 Cancerous growths around the vulva are pretty rare and usually painless, though your doctor will probably advise removal of a lump, especially if the swelling grows rapidly, causes pain or bleeding.
3 Fibroids in the womb are very common, almost exclusively innocent and are usually discovered on a routine internal examination as often they do not cause complaints even if they grow quite large.
4 They start as tiny seedlings, often grow very slowly, tend to enlarge in pregnancy and get smaller after the menopause.
5 Small fibroids that do not cause problems may need no

treatment, do not usually hamper your chances of getting pregnant and do not usually cause problems during pregnancy, though the likelihood of miscarriage may be slightly higher than normal.

6 Surgery may be indicated by an increase in the fibroids' size, by pain or excessively heavy periods.

7 The most satisfactory form of surgery for fibroids is to remove the whole womb containing the fibroids (hysterectomy).

8 If your doctor suspects that an internal swelling is coming from the ovary, you will probably be referred for a specialist opinion. This is because swellings of the ovary tend to cause more problems than fibroids, i.e. they can burst, or twist and become inflamed and there is always a small chance that an early cancer may be present.

9 Endometriosis is a fairly common condition often found by chance during investigations for pain or infertility. In the early stages medical treatment with special drugs is effective.

10 If the uterus and ovaries are extensively involved surgical treatment may be necessary. If you are anxious to conceive, surgery will be as conservative as possible. If your childbearing years are over, hysterectomy and removal of the ovaries should effect a permanent cure.

11 Removal of *one* ovary and tube should not reduce the chances of pregnancy.

5 Genital infections

During the reproductive life of a woman the genital organs are constantly being subjected to certain stresses from menstruation, pregnancy and sexual intercourse, and the delicate nature of the genital tissue makes infection a reasonably common occurrence. Inflammation may occur in any of the pelvic organs and by far the commonest presenting symptom is a vaginal discharge.

Vaginal discharge

Non-infective discharges

Vaginal discharge does not necessarily imply infection, as the walls of the vagina and the lining of the cervix constantly liberate a clear colourless fluid in most women. This normal discharge is particularly common in young girls who are approaching puberty, during pregnancy and at the time of ovulation midway between the periods. Women using the contraceptive Pill may notice an increase in discharge because the Pill contains the hormone oestrogen which makes the neck of the womb and the cells lining the vagina particularly moist. This discharge is colourless, clear and occasionally sticky. It should not cause an odour or be irritant. Although non-infective discharges usually require no treatment, if the fluid becomes excessive the doctor should be consulted so that a swab test can be taken.

Infective discharges

In the young girl who has not yet menstruated and in the older woman who has reached the menopause a yellowy discharge, sometimes with an unpleasant odour, is not unusual. This is because at the extremes of reproductive life the adult cells of the vagina are not sufficiently mature to keep the vagina moist and acid as the hormone oestrogen is not being produced by the ovaries. The result is that the vaginal walls become brittle and dry causing the cells lining the vagina to be shed in the form of a discharge. A swab test from the vagina should exclude a source of infection and treatment is usually by hormone cream or pessary.

During reproductive life inflammation of the vagina commonly occurs as a result of infection with two organisms. The first is called trichomonas vaginitis (TV) which causes a characteristic frothy, bubbly, green discharge, sometimes with an unpleasant odour, but generally no irritation. A simple swab test will demonstrate this organism and the treatment consists of taking a special antibiotic called Flagyl three times a day for ten days. Because the infection is sexually transmitted between partners it is best for the male to undertake a course of treatment as well. Apart from nuisance value there is no other significance to this sort of discharge, neither are there any serious consequences for either sex.

The other common type of discharge is quite different in appearance; the organism is a fungus called thrush or monilia, and it causes a white cheesy discharge with intense irritation and burning around the vulva and the vagina and sometimes scalding on passing urine. The thrush fungus is in fact a normal inhabitant of the vagina in many women and also lives quite peacefully in the mouth and intestines of men and women, causing no harm. Under certain circumstances the fungus will grow and multiply causing discharge and irritation, notably when the vagina has a sugary atmosphere in which the thrush organism thrives. This suitable environment is produced when there is an excess of oestrogen in the body, i.e. during pregnancy, in women taking the contraceptive Pill and if diabetes is present.

A flare-up of thrush infection can also occur following a prolonged course of antibiotics as the lining of the vagina becomes more susceptible.

The man may harbour the thrush fungus in the penis and urine but seldom realizes it. Infection can therefore be transmitted to the female during intercourse. There are a variety of treatments for vaginal thrush and these usually take the form of antibiotics, pessaries and creams inserted into the vagina for a week to ten days. Again this sort of discharge has no serious consequence but unfortunately tends to recur from time to time unless treatment is energetic. Recurrent thrush can be extremely irksome and not easy to cure. If recurrent courses of vaginal antibiotic do not eradicate the infection, treatment is directed towards changing the hormone environment of the vagina by advising a change of contraception if the Pill is being used, cleaning the neck of the womb if an erosion is present (see below) and washing the vagina with a strong antiseptic.

Rarely vaginal discharge is caused by a foreign body retained in the vagina such as a tampon that has inadvertently been overlooked, or part of a toy or small bead that a young girl has accidentally lodged in the vagina.

The neck of the womb or cervix is commonly the source of a vaginal discharge. A yellowish thick discharge, particularly heavy after childbirth or occurring in those on the Pill, usually arises from the cervix. There is no irritation or odour but the discharge may be quite profuse and cause considerable annoyance. This is usually due to a condition called a *cervical erosion* which simply means that the outside surface of the neck of the womb, which is normally covered by many layers of cells rather like the tip of the nose, has been rubbed away and replaced by much more delicate tissue which is contained within the canal of the neck of the womb. The cervix has a characteristic red appearance instead of the smooth skin-like surface normally present, and it is easy therefore to see how these new cells cause irritation and therefore discharge. If the discharge persists treatment consists either of touching the neck of the womb with an acid stick which is quite painless, or if the area of the neck of the womb that is involved is too large then admission to hospital is advised so that a full anaesthetic may be given and the neck of the womb treated a little more energetically by a small burner which destroys the surface cells and allows the new skin to grow over. For the first few days or maybe a week after this procedure the discharge in fact may increase or become slightly blood-stained as the cervix heals. As this sort of a discharge is sometimes made worse by the contraceptive Pill a temporary change of contraception may be advised.

A blood-stained discharge or bleeding that occurs *unassociated* with the menstrual cycle should always be reported to the doctor. It may be caused by the erosion that has already been discussed or possibly a small polyp arising from the neck of the womb; or in the older age group by an early growth which should be diagnosed and treated straight away.

Rarely, the body of the womb itself may be the source of a vaginal discharge. During reproductive life the commonest cause is again a foreign body in the womb such as an intra-uterine contraceptive device that causes irritation of the womb lining if allowed to remain in the uterus too long. In the later age group the cause is usually dryness or old-age of the skin of the lining of the womb, leading to shedding of the cells of the vagina and a discharge. Treatment consists of inserting hormone pessaries in the vagina which help to restore the tone of the tissues and render them less brittle. A yellow or blood-stained discharge that occurs for the first time after the periods have ceased must be reported to the doctor soon as occasionally this is the first symptom of a small growth inside the body of the womb.

Soreness and irritation of the vagina

Because the skin of the vulva and vagina is particularly sensitive it is not unusual for these sites to be a source of irritation or itchiness. Irritation is commonly associated with one of the vaginal discharges that have already been discussed, particularly that caused by the fungus organism thrush. If there is no discharge and the symptoms become distressing medical advice should be sought because further investigation may be indicated. Certain diseases of the skin such as eczema or dermatitis may cause a rash as well as irritation, and sometimes this complaint is the first manifestation of a general disease process such as diabetes. It may be that a little leakage of urine that sometimes occurs in patients who have a dropping of the womb or prolapse may continually irritate the delicate tissues of the vulva and vagina; or irritation may arise from the back passage or rectum due to piles or infestation with worms. In the older woman, persistent irritation of the vulva may occur with patchy white discoloration of the skin. This condition is one of a group of skin disorders occurring principally in those past the menopause and should be reported to the doctor as a diagnosis must be made before treatment is advised. This is done by removing a small piece of skin for microscopical examination.

Poor hygiene, woollen or nylon underclothes or the application of certain antiseptic solutions or creams may cause irritation and worsen the existing condition. Those who have a predisposition to allergies such as asthma and hay fever may complain of irritation around the vulva.

One of the problems with the vaginal itchiness is that it causes a desire to scratch which leads to further irritation so a vicious circle is set up often with an emotional element. Sometimes no obvious cause for irritation can be found after detailed investigation and the only treatment, which can sometimes be very painstaking, is breaking the circle. This implies confidence and a sympathetic understanding by the medical practitioner and frank discussion about possible underlying sexual frustration.

Infection of the fallopian tubes (salpingitis)

Of all genital infections involvement of the fallopian tubes is probably the most serious. This is not only because this condition can be extremely painful and distressing but also because fertility may be impaired. Unfortunately, infection of the fallopian tubes is a common condition and because of their extreme delicacy the tubes may easily become blocked, preventing transfer of the fertilized egg.

Why does this condition occur?

Just as the advantage of the female genital tract having an opening to the outside may allow early detection of a cancer, so the disadvantage allows certain organisms which may cause infection to enter the vagina and climb through the cervix into the womb and into the fallopian tubes. This form of ascending infection will occur more frequently after childbirth or after a miscarriage or when a pregnancy has been terminated. Occasionally the fallopian tubes may become infected by direct spread from neighbouring structures inside the abdomen which are themselves inflamed. The fallopian tube, particularly on the right, is very close to the appendix and inflammation of the appendix may spread directly to involve the fallopian tube. In the days when tuberculosis was common the fallopian tubes were implicated as a secondary source of infection in a high percentage of cases. Happily, with modern treatment and virtual eradication of this disease in the Western world this is no longer much of a problem.

The main complaints of salpingitis include feeling unwell and feverish, lower abdominal pain on both sides and a particularly offensive vaginal discharge. There is often quite a severe frontal headache. If the diagnosis is made early and antibiotic treatment immediately started there is a good chance that no impairment of tubal functions and fertility will result and the prognosis is good. Very rarely will any surgical intervention be necessary provided a diagnosis can be made with surety. If the diagnosis is in doubt or there is no response to antibiotics then examination under anaesthetic may be needed together with an exploratory operation.

Sometimes acute inflammation of the tubes recurs and in principle the same treatment applies.

Occasionally recurrent attacks of inflammation of the fallopian tubes recur in later life causing long-standing inflammation. Periods may become heavy and painful, and the pelvic organs tender. There is often low backache and sexual intercourse is painful. If this condition continues to recur after child-bearing years are over removal of the tubes may be indicated. Because the organisms have to pass through the neck of the womb and into the body of the womb before they attack the fallopian tubes, some surgeons will suggest that removal of the womb and ovaries is necessary as well.

Venereal disease

The word 'venereal' means relating to sexual intercourse. Venereal disease is a term used to describe a group of infections which are passed from person to person through sexual contact. Strictly speaking trichomonas and thrush (see earlier this chapter) are therefore venereal diseases though they are not generally referred to in the same context as the two serious venereal diseases gonorrhoea and syphilis. These disorders have little in common except that they are always passed on by sexual contact. This is because the causative organisms usually live in the infected person's genital organs or in some place where they have been placed by sexual activity, and to infect another they have to enter the body through an orifice. Sexual activity gives them this chance.

Gonorrhoea

This condition is by far the commoner of the two and is still spreading alarmingly fast among people of all ages and social classes. Roughly 65,000 cases of gonorrhoea are reported per year in the United Kingdom. As with syphilis there was a post-war peak in incidence of the disease but during the last ten years this peak has now been exceeded, with a greater rise seen among women than among men.

Gonorrhoea is caused by a bacterium that thrives in the warm moist lining of the urethra or water channel, the rectum, and the mouth and neck of the womb – the cervix. Though it is normally only passed on by sexual contact the unborn child of a mother who has untreated gonorrhoea may be born with the disease. Contrary to popular rumour it cannot be acquired by contact with objects such as a contaminated towel or a toilet seat. One of the problems is that frequently there are no symptoms, and it has been estimated that between 70 to 80 per cent of cases in women occur without their having any awareness of it.

Symptoms in the female

Within five to seven days of sexual contact with an infected person an offensive yellow discharge occurs together with pain and frequency on passing urine. Treatment at this stage is completely successful, but if delayed the bacteria will spread into the uterus and along the fallopian tubes causing inflammation and blockage, with possible sterility. It is therefore essential for a woman who has these symptoms to present herself to her doctor or to a local clinic with some urgency. The diagnosis will be made by taking swabs from the water channel and the neck of the womb and the anal canal where the bacteria first are harboured and they are then identified with a microscope. Contrary to former belief there is no specific blood test that can make the diagnosis positively and the organism has to be grown on swab tests.

Treatment consists of large doses of antibiotics, usually one of the penicillin group of drugs, and it is important that a doctor who works in venereal clinics be notified as contacts must be traced and treated in order to prevent spread of the condition. Sometimes there may be considerable delay between sexual contact and the onset of symptoms so that the woman may present for the first time with pain in the abdomen due to tubal inflammation.

Symptoms in the male

About 10 per cent of men have no symptoms at all and are oblivious to the condition. For the remaining, pain on urination, discomfort inside the penis or a discharge from the penis tip should suggest immediate consultation with a doctor. The incubation period in men, in other words the time between sexual contact and the onset of symptoms, is usually under a week but it can be as long as a month. The diagnosis is again made by culturing the organism after taking swabs from the discharge and treatment should begin immediately.

Syphilis

This is a far more awesome condition which is often hard to detect in the woman. It is caused by a small organism shaped like a corkscrew that is able to twist and burrow its way through tiny breaks in the skin. The incubation period is usually between fourteen and twenty-eight days but is sometimes as long as ninety days after sexual intercourse. Unlike gonorrhoea the disease process is slow and insidious and if untreated it progresses through three stages. The first two are infectious, following which spontaneous healing usually occurs, after this there may be a long latent period where the disease lies dormant. In about 30 per cent of untreated patients late disease of the heart or central nervous system, or other organs, ultimately develops, which can lead to difficulty with walking, destructive changes in the joints, sometimes even incontinence of the bladder and occasionally a gradual loss of brain function resulting in psychosis and insanity, with impaired memory, defective judgement, depression and delusions.

Symptoms
The first symptom may be a small sore which appears on one of the lips of the vulva. Usually painless, this sore heals itself within six to ten weeks. Similarly the male partner may complain of a sore on the penis. Sometimes small swellings appear in the groin which are inflamed lymph glands. If the organism gets into the bloodstream, a non-itchy skin rash may appear anywhere on the body from the scalp down to and including the soles of the feet, on the chest, back or arms and characteristically it disappears as fast as it arrives. These symptoms usually disappear without treatment after three weeks or may last nine months, but if untreated the condition remains hidden in the body and may reappear some twenty to thirty years later. Usually after about two years the woman ceases to be infectious though syphilis can still be passed to a baby she bears.

Diagnosis of the condition is not easy to make. A scraping is usually taken from the initial sore in the hope of growing the organism responsible. There are also special blood tests available but expert advice should be sought from the practitioner or a local venereology clinic if there is the slightest suspicion of contact. Treatment consists of large doses of antibiotics with careful follow-up and the tracing of contacts.

Genital herpes (cold sores)

This condition is caused by a virus similar to the commoner type of condition which causes sore blisters around the chest called shingles. It lies in the skin inactive for long periods but when it becomes activated it causes a genital or anal sore that usually weeps a colourless fluid and forms a scab. Most genital herpes infections are caused by contact with the virus during sexual intercourse. The condition causes swollen painful blisters or blister-like eruptions around the vulva. Unfortunately, like so many virus conditions there is no specific treatment, but discomfort can be relieved by applying special ointments, one of the most helpful called Herpid. The condition is self-limiting and tends to be related to emotion and anxiety.

Points to note

1 A vaginal discharge does not necessarily imply infection. A non-irritant colourless discharge which can become quite heavy during a pregnancy or if you are taking the contraceptive Pill is not unusual.
2 A white scaly discharge which makes you want to scratch is usually due to thrush. Treatment with antibiotic pessaries is generally effective.
3 A frothy green discharge with an unpleasant odour may be due to trichomonas vaginitis (TV). Though often acquired through sexual contact, a short course of antibiotics for you and your partner should cure the infection, with no lasting harmful effects.
4 Any discharge that comes after the menopause, particularly if it is yellow or tinged with blood, should be reported. Usually this is due to simple dryness of the skin which can be cured

by hormone creams. Occasionally it may be the first sign of a polyp or early growth.

5 Provided that inflammation of the fallopian tubes (salpingitis) is treated early there should be no impairment of future fertility.

6 A thick yellow discharge with scalding on passing urine occurring for the first time a few days after sexual intercourse may be the first sign of gonorrhoea. A simple swab test will confirm the diagnosis and prompt treatment should effect a complete cure. Where possible both partners should be treated with antibiotics to prevent reinfection.

6 Urinary problems

Urinary complaints and infections occur more commonly in women than in men because there is a very close connection between the vaginal passage and the bladder and also because the channel leading from the bladder to the exterior (urethra) is extremely short, about 3 cm in length. For this reason any organisms or bacteria that are present in the genital region can easily gain entrance into the bladder and if they are not washed away by the urine in the bladder these bacteria may climb up the channel leading from the kidneys to the bladder (ureter) and cause infection in the kidneys.

Pregnancy and childbirth contribute to infection as the urinary channels widen under hormonal influence, encouraging urine to collect and stagnate.

Frequent and painful urination

Passing urine at more frequent intervals than usual is often the first symptom of an infection and this may or may not be accompanied by burning or scalding. Sometimes frequency of urination is caused by pressure on the bladder by an enlargement of the womb or cyst of an ovary leading to discomfort in the abdomen or a recognizable swelling. Because the genital and urinary systems are so closely connected, inflammation of the fallopian tubes or the neck of the womb may indirectly cause urinary symptoms. Nervousness and habit may lead to frequent urination which is usually not accompanied by any discomfort or burning but tends to be self-perpetuating. Apart from infection in the urinary system burning on urination may be caused by an infection in the neighbouring vaginal tissues such as thrush infection or more rarely by a stone in the bladder or a small tumour in the urethral channel.

Painful urination can occur shortly after intercourse and is most commonly the result of bruising to the urethral passage. The penis may rub against the floor of the urethra and bladder, particularly if there is insufficient vaginal lubrication or a tight vaginal opening. This is common with advancing age as the vaginal walls become thin and inelastic and unable to stretch during intercourse, making the neighbouring urinary structures more vulnerable to injury or inflammation. This often distressing symptom can be considerably improved by using a bland lubricating cream during intercourse, or a hormone cream.

Frequency of urination or scalding that persists should be reported to the doctor as a general examination and investigation of a specimen of urine will often demonstrate a cause that can easily be treated.

Cystitis

Strictly this word means inflammation of the bladder but it is often used to indicate an infection of the urine which may form in any part of the urinary system and not the bladder alone. It is estimated that 75 per cent of women will have an attack of cystitis at some stage in their lives and some of the reasons for this common condition have already been described.

Usually there is an intense *desire* to pass water every few minutes though very little urine appears. An intense burning sensation accompanies urination and occasionally the urine may be tinged with blood. There may also be pain in the lower abdomen and the urine may have a strong smell.

The first test a doctor will want is a specimen of urine because it is very important to treat cystitis with the correct antibiotic and in order to do this the laboratory will have to examine the urine to find out which organism is responsible. It is helpful to drink some water before seeing the doctor so that the bladder fills and a specimen can be obtained. Because many harmless bacteria live around the urethral opening it is important that the doctor receives as clean a specimen of urine as possible. The entrance to the vagina should be swabbed and a sample of urine taken halfway through urination (midstream specimen of urine). The pathologist will be able to pinpoint the bacteria responsible for the infection within twenty-four to forty-eight hours. Occasionally one or two specimens show no evidence of infection though symptoms persist; further investigations by means of urine tests, blood tests and X-rays are then required.

Treatment

Once the bacteria responsible for the infection have been identified treatment is started with the appropriate antibiotic which is usually taken for a minimum of five days. A high fluid intake is helpful in keeping the urine well diluted and the symptoms are usually relieved within twenty-four to forty-eight hours of starting treatment. Here a word of caution: it is important to continue the antibiotic treatment for as long as the doctor prescribes, however tempting it is to stop treatment within a couple of days when the symptoms may have disappeared. The infection can still be present and premature interruption of treatment will only cause a further flare-up. The doctor may require a second specimen of urine after ten days to make sure that the urine is now sterile.

During an attack of cystitis it may be comforting to have a day in bed and take soluble aspirin every four hours to relieve the pain. Other helpful measures include a high fluid intake, a teaspoon of bicarbonate of soda which removes the acidity of the urine, and warmth from a hot water bottle.

Honeymoon cystitis

Sometimes cystitis occurs only after sexual intercourse. Known as 'honeymoon cystitis' because attacks invariably start early in married life, this occurs because the urethral channel is extremely short and intercourse tends to work bacteria up into the bladder.

It is helpful if both partners wash carefully before intercourse, and if the vaginal passage is particularly dry the vagina should be lubricated with a bland jelly. It is also useful to pass urine soon after intercourse in order to flush out any bacteria that might have ascended into the urethra. Although these symptoms of cystitis are transient it is important to obtain a specimen of urine to exclude infection.

Burning on passing urine with frequency following sexual intercourse is not always caused by a specific bacterium and there remains a group of women, often in the latter age group, who continue to have these distressing symptoms for which no cause is found when the urine is examined. The most probable explanation is the lack of smoothness and elasticity of the vagina and urethra which occurs around the menopause as the hormone oestrogen, normally responsible for this tone, gradually diminishes. Treatment is often unsatisfactory but the principles involve cleanliness before and after intercourse, use of a lubricating jelly together with local application of a hormone cream. Relief from cystitis following intercourse can sometimes be obtained by taking a short course of antibiotics after sex.

If cystitis recurs frequently or if the symptoms of passing urine repeatedly in the absence of an infection persist, further investigations of the urinary tract are undertaken. This involves urine and blood tests, a special X-ray which demonstrates the urinary tract and the kidneys, and possible admission to hospital for an examination under anaesthetic and visualization of the lining of the bladder with a torch (cystoscopy) to exclude any of the rarer causes, such as a bladder stone or abnormality of the kidney.

Incontinence

Incontinence means that there is an inability to retain urine in the bladder which will result in constant dribbling and leakage. Although this is a very worrying complaint there are certain times in a woman's life when mild forms of incontinence occur normally and resolve without any treatment.

Bed-wetting is a form of incontinence and occurs commonly in young children. Blame should not be attached either to the parents or to the child for in the great majority of instances bed-wetting will cease quite spontaneously as puberty approaches. The cause is probably an immaturity of the normal control reflex that passes from the brain to the nerves of the bladder and in some children this reflex, initiating the desire to urinate, is not fully developed into the adult state. However reassuring this explanation may be it is not easy for the parents of a bed-wetting child to cope with the endless changing of soiled bed linen and the frustration of the child herself which often manifests itself in a 'couldn't care less' attitude, though in truth there is often considerable turmoil in the child's mind about the problem.

Most girls are dry at night between the ages of two and five, though this age limit is variable. If incontinence at night continues after seven, medical advice should be sought if for no other reason than to obtain reassurance. Although bed-wetting is usually unassociated with any disease in the child, the possibility of infection in the urine must be excluded first.

Treatment consists of a sympathetic understanding of the problem in the knowledge that in the great majority of instances bed-wetting will resolve itself quite spontaneously by the age of ten or eleven. It is often helpful to teach the child to hold urine in the bladder for increasing periods of time during the day, and to avoid bedtime drinks. Some doctors consider that bed-wetting may be improved dramatically by correct nappy training and mild sedative drugs, though it is often the mother rather than the child who benefits most from tranquilliser treatment! If incontinence persists it may be worth seeking advice about bed-wetting alarm systems which consist of a thin sheet in which is wound a sensitive wire which leads to an alarm; when a drop of urine touches the lower sheet a current sets off a bell, immediately waking the child. This device often helps to educate the reflex of urination and further information can be obtained from local health authority child clinics or the family doctor. It is most unusual for bed-wetting to continue into the teens but rarely it lasts until the age of about twenty before resolving.

Leakage of urine can occur for the first time during a pregnancy and this is due to a combination of hormone factors and slight sagging of the bladder (see Chapter 7). Similarly this symptom may occur for the first time after the menopause and treatment is discussed in Chapter 12.

Sometimes, however, the ability to retain urine in the bladder may be impaired for the first time in the younger woman to such an extent that urine leaks from the bladder on exertion, in other words after coughing, sneezing, running for a bus or even turning over in bed at night. Doctors call this symptom *stress* incontinence because it only occurs during some exertion and not at rest. This is often the first symptom of a prolapsed womb and the management of it will be described in Chapter 7.

Rarely, a form of leakage called *true* incontinence exists, when the woman wets herself constantly without any knowledge of this happening and without any stress or exertion. This symptom may occur in children born with certain abnormalities of the control of urination due to a spinal cord deformity or in the older woman with advanced cancer of the womb which has spread to the bladder.

Finally, there is *urge* incontinence. Perhaps incontinence here is not a good word because strictly this means that there is an intense desire to void so that the woman finds herself running to and from the lavatory constantly with the unpleasant feeling that she may not get there in time, though leakage of urine rarely occurs. This symptom may occur with cystitis, but may also occur in the absence of infection, often in later life. Here the problem usually lies with the bladder itself and its muscle tone, and once the diagnosis is made treatment is usually by tablets which relax the muscle of the bladder or sometimes by a small operation whereby the urethral channel leading from the bladder to the exterior is stretched under general anaesthetic.

It can be seen that incontinence of urine is a complicated complaint with a number of causes and this is why time spent at the initial consultation with the doctor is so important. In order to make a provisional diagnosis the doctor must know what type of incontinence he is dealing with. Does leakage of urine only occur following stress or exertion? Is there an intense desire to go to the lavatory often? Does incontinence occur at night?

Does scalding or burning accompany leakage of urine ? Accurate answers to these questions can be invaluable in detecting the different types of incontinence of urine and go a long way towards correct treatment.

Blood in the urine

Normal urine is either quite clear or slightly yellow-coloured and contains no blood. If the urine becomes blood-stained together with symptoms of scalding during voiding this is probably due to cystitis which is by far the commonest cause of this symptom. Occasionally the urine is pink or red-stained and there are no associated urinary symptoms, when the cause may again be urinary infection and a specimen of urine will confirm the diagnosis. However, painless blood in the urine must be investigated further as rarely there may be a stone or a polyp present or a growth in the urinary channel. In the young woman isolated instances of blood in the urine can occur and following investigations no definite diagnosis is made and the condition does not recur. In the later age group, however, this symptom must be reported soon to the doctor so that he can arrange referral to a gynaecologist or urologist.

Inability to pass urine

To complete the picture of urinary disorders brief mention must be made of the rare complaint of being unable to pass urine (retention of urine). Although the urge to urinate is intense the bladder cannot empty with the result that it fills with more urine causing intense abdominal discomfort and a swelling in the lower part of the abdomen. The discomfort can be relieved immediately by the passage of a catheter or tube passed through the urethral channel allowing the urine to drain out of the bladder.

Why does this happen?
Immediately after childbirth or after some surgical operations it is quite common for the bladder not to empty properly and it

may be a few hours before spontaneous urination occurs. Usually this symptom rights itself before the need for a catheter arises. Rarely, retention of urine is caused by a large swelling in one of the pelvic organs which presses on the bladder and alters its position so that the outflow of urine is obstructed. Similarly, in the first three months of pregnancy the womb that is enlarging with the developing embryo presses on the urethral channel and bladder under certain circumstances and prevents normal emptying (see Chapter 7).

Finally, inability to pass urine may be a nervous manifestation caused by anxiety or emotional upsets.

Points to note

1 Because the opening to the urinary channel is very close to the vaginal passage, any bacteria present in the vagina can find their way easily into the bladder and up to the kidneys causing infection of the urine. This is particularly likely to occur during pregnancy or after childbirth.

2 A urinary infection will probably make you want to pass water more frequently, often with a burning and stinging sensation. You may also get an intense desire to empty your bladder or a feeling of incomplete emptying.

3 Cystitis really means an inflammation of the bladder. Because different organisms can be responsible for infections it is important that a specimen of urine is tested before treatment so that the correct antibiotic which is sensitive to the organism is prescribed. Though you may feel better within 24 to 48 hours of treatment you should carry on with the whole course of treatment as prescribed by your doctor. Premature interruption of treatment will only partially cure the infection and it may return.

4 Bed-wetting in childhood is not a disease. However embarrassing and unpleasant the chores of continual changing of soiled bed linen may be, scolding and reprimand are seldom effective. It is unusual for bed-wetting to continue after puberty.

5 Leakage of small amounts of urine often occur during pregnancy, particularly following some exertion such as running,

coughing, sneezing. If this continues after childbirth, or gets worse, go and see your doctor. You may have a minor degree of dropping of the womb or prolapse that will respond to muscle strengthening exercises or perhaps require a small operation.

6 Don't ignore blood-stained urine. Probably it is due to a urinary infection but occasionally there may be a small polyp or growth in the bladder. A visit to the doctor should put your mind at rest.

7 Abnormal positions of the womb

The dropped womb (prolapse)

In order to understand what is meant by this condition imagine the uterus to be suspended in the lower part of the abdomen by various supports called ligaments and muscles which are responsible for holding it in the correct position – rather like a tent supported by guy ropes. If these guy ropes become overstretched or frayed because of wear and tear then the tent will gradually become unstable and begin to sag or even drop completely to the ground. In the same way, if the supports of the uterus become weak the womb will descend downwards into the vaginal passage and in an extreme case the leading part of the womb – the cervix – may drop so far that it is actually visible and noticed by the patient as a lump at the entrance to the vagina.

What causes this?
By far the commonest cause is the stretching of the tissues by the passage of the baby through the birth canal during childbirth. In order to be able to push the baby's head through the pelvis the mother must use her pelvic muscles to their maximum ability and this will inevitably cause some stretching and looseness of the tissues. If the mother starts to push too early or if the baby is large and the mother has to push for too long then the supporting tissues may become excessively stretched. It can be seen that the correct management of the expulsive stage of labour by the attending doctor or midwife is crucially important in the prevention of a prolapse of the womb. This overstretching can be prevented either by a small cut in the back wall of the vagina

which allows more room for the baby's head to emerge (episiotomy), or sometimes the doctor will help the baby's head out with forceps. In countries where little help is available for mothers in labour, extreme degrees of prolapse are quite common in young women.

Whereas the great majority of women who have a prolapsed womb have had children, the condition sometimes occurs for the first time after the change of life in a woman who has not conceived. Here the weakness of the supports is not caused by stretching but by the natural process of old age which becomes pronounced because the ovaries stop producing oestrogen which is partly responsible for the normal elastic tone of these supports. Very rarely a young child may have this symptom due to a congenital abnormality or even absence of some of these supporting tissues.

A sagging womb will be worsened by obesity, a chronic smoker's cough, and an occupation that involves heavy lifting.

What are the symptoms?

This will really depend on what part of the womb and its surrounding structures have dropped and the degree of slackness. The womb is very closely attached to the bladder in front, and the back passage or rectum behind, and therefore these structures will drop with the womb causing symptoms involving the urinary system and the bowels.

The commonest complaint is the inability to retain urine on exertion. This is called stress incontinence and means that the woman wets herself when she coughs, sneezes, laughs, runs, or sometimes when she turns over in bed at night. Why this actually happens is obscure but part of the problem rests with the fact that the bladder descends with the womb in the condition of prolapse and the water channel leading from the bladder to the outside (urethra), instead of making an angle with the bladder, is in a straight line, so that any expulsive effort will shoot urine out of the water channel and soil underclothes. Sometimes there is an urge to empty the bladder very frequently but only a small amount of urine is passed with a feeling that the bladder is not fully empty. This is called urgency of urination and is fully discussed in Chapter 6. Sometimes prolapse causes recurrent urinary infections or cystitis with frequent urination by day and night, and scalding.

Just as the bladder drops down with the womb so the rectum can prolapse as well, and women may find difficulty in emptying the bowels completely.

If the womb descends far down the vaginal passage a swelling may be noticed at the vaginal entrance and a feeling of 'something coming down' – particularly at the end of the day – accompanied by backache and heaviness low down in the pelvis. The swelling may be either the bladder which has dropped down in front of the womb or the neck of the womb itself which has dropped so far down that it appears at or outside the entrance to the vagina.

What treatment can be given?

Many women who have had children will have some degree of slackness of the supporting tissues which may give rise to very few complaints. If a doctor notices a small degree of prolapse on examination which is not giving rise to any trouble then no treatment is necessary. Much can be done to prevent the prolapse by good obstetric care during delivery and by encouraging early activity soon after childbirth together with education in tightening the pelvic muscles during the lying-in period. Here the skill of the physiotherapist is of great value and most obstetric units have the services of a physiotherapist who helps in the preparation of childbirth and also with the post-natal care of the mother.

Although women who have a mild dropping can be taught to strengthen their own muscles to a certain extent, by tightening and loosening the muscles of the buttock for a few seconds, thus attempting to stop passing urine in midstream, if symptoms are severe or the degree of prolapse pronounced then more active management may be needed.

This usually takes the form of a surgical repair of the parts of the prolapse that have sagged so that the pelvic organs are re-suspended in their normal position. The type of surgery and extent will depend on the degree of prolapse and whether any future pregnancies are contemplated. Although there is no absolute contra-indication to surgical repair of a dropped womb, if further children are desired it is best to leave surgery until child-bearing years are over because much of the good work may be undone by the stress of another pregnancy and labour.

If the neck of the womb has dropped the surgeon may remove it as a part of the repair operation or it may be suggested that the whole of the womb is removed from the vagina (vaginal hysterectomy) to prevent the possibility of the condition recurring.

Some gynaecologists prefer to repair the dropped womb and others to remove it. The latter procedure is more commonly adopted in the older patient, particularly if it is necessary to remove the womb anyway for other reasons. It is usual also to tighten the back part of the vagina, particularly if this part is bulging forwards or if it is noticed that the vagina is wider than usual and consequently intercourse not so satisfying.

If surgery is refused, or contra-indicated because of a disabling condition that prevents a general anaesthetic, a pessary can be fitted in the vagina. These pessaries are circular appliances made of rubber or plastic which should be unnoticed as they lie in position. When the correct size is chosen the pessary fits snugly between the front and back walls of the vagina preventing the

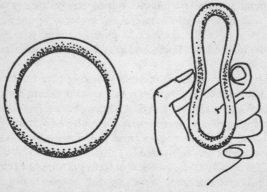

The ring pessary inserted into the vagina for a prolapsed uterus

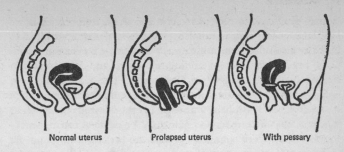

Normal uterus   Prolapsed uterus   With pessary

Normal uterus, prolapsed uterus, and with pessary

womb from prolapsing downwards. This treatment does not cure the dropped womb, merely supporting the womb temporarily. The pessary may occasionally fail to hold the prolapsed womb in position and needs to be changed every few months. It may cause an irritating and sometimes odorous discharge, or even abrasions on the surrounding vaginal wall, interfering with normal intercourse.

Nowadays, with advanced anaesthetic techniques, age in itself is no bar to surgery, and although the vaginal pessary can be a real blessing for some who do obtain symptomatic relief many women in their seventies or eighties are having their prolapses surgically corrected and are in far better shape afterwards.

The tilted womb (retroverted womb)

The normal position of the womb is at 90° to the vagina so that the body of the womb is bent *forwards*. In about 15 per cent of women for no reason whatsoever the womb is at 90° to the vagina again but bent *backwards*, and this is called retroversion. The fact that the womb is bent backwards usually has no significance unless it is the cause of a gynaecological complaint.

After childbirth the womb is normally retroverted temporarily and it is quite common at the post-natal examination six weeks after delivery that this position is maintained. In the majority of instances, retroversion will cause no complaints and is a purely incidental finding so no treatment is necessary. Sometimes, however, the womb that is tilted backwards is tender and fixed so that any attempt to move it causes pain during the examination. This occurs with long-standing infection and the condition known as endometriosis (see Chapter 4). The womb may also be pulled into a backward position by a swelling or tumour in the womb itself or possibly by a prolapse. If the womb becomes fixed in a position of retroversion pain may be noticed during intercourse. This is not so much because the penis impinges on the womb itself but because the ovaries which lie on either side of the womb fall down into the back of the pelvis because the womb is retroverted and pressure on the ovaries during intercourse will cause discomfort.

There are two main indications for repositioning the retroverted womb: (1) when it is causing severe pain during inter-

Replacing a retroverted uterus.

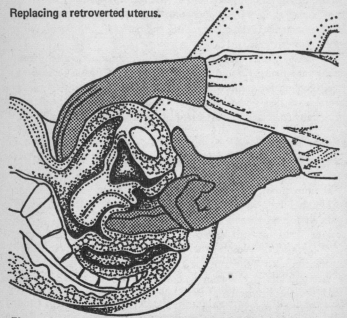

Fingers in the vagina pushing the uterus forward.

Replacing a retroverted uterus.

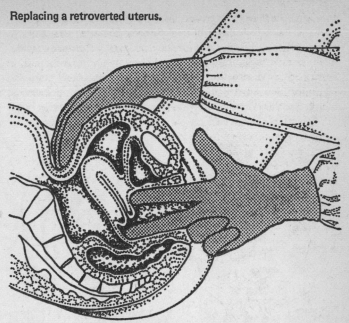

Outside hand catching the uterus.

course, all other causes for this pain having been excluded; and
(2) in certain cases of infertility and frequent early miscarriages.
It used to be thought that the position of the cervix of the retroverted uterus gave it less contact with the pool of semen deposited during intercourse and therefore decreased chances of conception, though it is doubtful if this is really so, and although
opinion is divided there is little proof that a retroverted uterus
increases the likelihood of miscarriage either.

Placing the womb in its upright position

There are two ways in which this can be done. If the womb can
be moved from side to side during internal examination, the
doctor may be able to replace it simply in the clinic by pushing
on the neck of the womb and bringing the body of it forward,
though if this can be done easily the womb is likely to fall back

into its retroverted position again soon afterwards. If the womb is fixed in a backward position and causes pain during intercourse and during examination, the same procedure may be possible under a light general anaesthetic. Once repositioned, a pessary inserted into the vagina for a few weeks may stabilize the womb and keep it upright. After six weeks the pessary is removed to see whether the womb remains upright or falls back

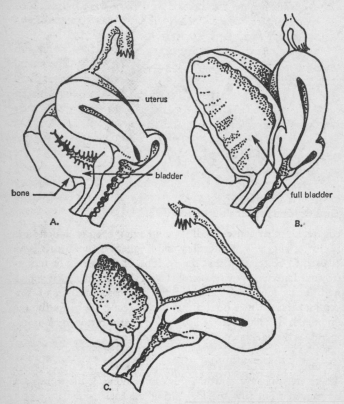

The 'normal' and 'retroverted' uterus showing
 A. how the uterus normally lies in the pelvis;
 B. how it may move when the bladder fills; and
 C. a retroverted uterus

again. If no pain during intercourse has been experienced with the pessary *in situ* and pain returns immediately after its removal because the womb has dropped backwards then it may be necessary to stitch the womb permanently in an upward position; this is done by a small operation through the abdomen whereby two of the supporting ropes or ligaments keeping the uterus upright are shortened. If the womb is retroverted because of associated disease such as infection or endometriosis or fibroids then the treatment of the condition will cure the symptoms and removal of the womb (hysterectomy) may be indicated.

There is one other instance when a retroverted womb can cause problems and this is during early pregnancy. The womb often points backwards in the first few weeks of pregnancy and gradually bends upwards as it grows so that by about fourteen weeks the uterus is usually upright and can be felt quite easily as a swelling in the abdomen. Occasionally the uterus does not come forward but remains tilted backwards. As it enlarges, the womb may press on the bladder making it impossible for the woman to pass water, and the bladder will have to be emptied by a catheter or tube. Relief is immediate and the catheter is usually left draining the bladder for twenty-four hours. Once withdrawn normal urination recurs spontaneously.

Points to note

1 Minor degrees of prolapse are common after childbirth and often respond to muscle strengthening exercises alone.
2 The first complaint is often leakage of urine after exertion (stress incontinence). If you are unable to run, dance or exert yourself without wetting your pants go and see the doctor. Stress incontinence is effectively cured by a minor operation.
3 If the whole womb sags into the vaginal passage, giving rise to a feeling of 'something coming down', you may need a full repair operation or removal of the womb. As a temporary measure a plastic ring may be inserted into the vaginal canal which holds up the womb.
4 Surgical operations for prolapse that repair the dropped

uterus do not necessarily prohibit further pregnancies but it is usual to defer surgery until you have finished your family as childbirth will put some strain on the supports of the womb, encouraging a recurrence of weakness.

5 The majority of operations for prolapse are done through the vagina and as a result the passage may be slightly shortened. Because the vagina is capable of stretching there should be no problem with intercourse. In fact many find sex more satisfying because the muscles supporting the vagina are deliberately tightened during the operation.

6 Occasionally a prolapse may recur. This is partly due to the fact that gravity tends to encourage the womb and its supports to drop down. Overweight, excessive heavy lifting and a chronic cough are other factors which encourage a recurrence.

7 A retroverted or backward-facing uterus is usually an incidental finding often causing no complaints and may not need treatment. Replacement of the uterus into the upright position may be recommended if intercourse is painful.

8 Contraception

Pregnancy will occur if healthy semen enters the woman's vagina, finds suitable conditions in the vaginal passage to live, if the sperm travel into the womb and down the fallopian tube and fertilization of the egg takes place, and if the womb provides a satisfactory bed for the fertilized egg to implant and grow. The deliberate prevention of a pregnancy may therefore be achieved if any of these conditions are altered or interrupted.

Attitudes have changed dramatically over the last ten to fifteen years, and thanks to the pioneering work of the Family Planning Association and similar advisory centres there is now a wide range of effective methods of preventing pregnancy. The correct method for any couple will depend on a number of factors, including individual suitability, degree of effectiveness, and emotional and cultural attitudes. Advice about family planning can be obtained from the family doctor or family planning clinics and since 1974 this service has been completely free for all women in this country.

Withdrawal (interrupted intercourse)

This is one of the oldest and simplest methods of birth control whereby the penis is withdrawn from the vagina just before the ejaculation of sperm. Although practised by many couples this method of contraception is often thought to be unsatisfactory because of the frustration of both partners and the fact that occasionally sperm deposited on the outer lips of the vulva may gain access to the vagina and gain entrance into the cervix.

The rhythm method (safe period)

This method of contraception is particularly practised by Roman Catholics who are unable to rely upon mechanical, chemical or other methods. Intercourse is planned to take place in the non-fertile phases of the menstrual cycle and depends on three facts. Firstly, ovulation only occurs once every cycle and the egg will only survive for about 36 hours; secondly, ovulation usually occurs 12 to 14 days before the first day of the next period; and thirdly, sperm can only survive for about 72 hours after ejaculation from the penis.

The rhythm method is only about 70 per cent effective and the main reason for the high failure rate is that ovulation does not necessarily occur exactly at the same time in the middle of each menstrual cycle even if the woman has regular periods. The timing of ovulation can be predicted by the rise in temperature that occurs after the egg has been shed (see Chapter 11). As the timing of ovulation can vary in each cycle, temperature recording should be taken daily for at least six months before a definite pattern can be established. The success of this method depends on a high degree of motivation by both partners.

Mechnical means of preventing sperm gaining access to the neck of the womb are the most widely used methods of contraception throughout the world and although their popularity has fluctuated since the introduction of more sophisticated techniques this method of family planning remains extremely effective and harmless.

The sheath

A sheath or condom (french letter; durex) is placed over the erect penis before intercourse so that during ejaculation the sperms remain inside the sheath and do not enter the vaginal passage. Originally used by Roman soldiers in order to prevent infection from venereal disease, this is the commonest contraceptive in use today. Modern sheaths cause no allergic reactions and should only be used once. Care should be taken to ensure that the condom does not come off the penis after ejaculation before withdrawing from the partner.

The chief disadvantage is interruption of love-making as the sheath has to be put on the erect penis. Sheaths can burst but this is extremely uncommon and if pregnancy results from this method it is usually due to incorrect use rather than a hole in the sheath. For complete safety against pregnancy it is better to combine the sheath with a special cream which is placed in the vagina and which will kill off any sperm that do happen to remain there after the sheath has been removed. The sheath may also provide some protection against sexually transmitted diseases.

The diaphragm

Invented in 1882, the common type of diaphragm was first marketed by a Dutch firm, hence the popular name – Dutch

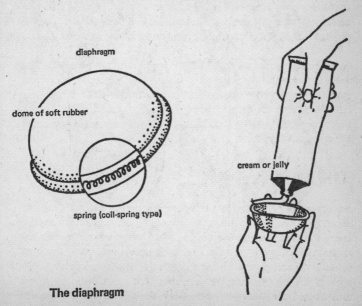

diaphragm

dome of soft rubber

spring (coil-spring type)

cream or jelly

The diaphragm

Cap. This is the commonest type of mechanical contraceptive used by women and consists of a soft rubber diaphragm with a coiled spring around the rim. Available in different sizes, an

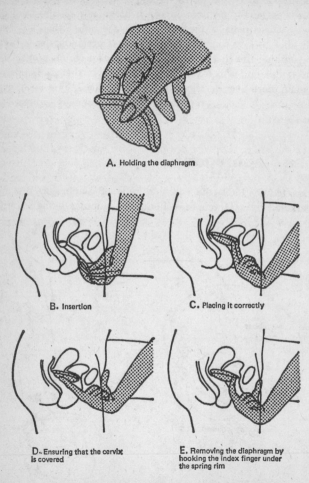

A. Holding the diaphragm

B. Insertion

C. Placing it correctly

D. Ensuring that the cervix is covered

E. Removing the diaphragm by hooking the index finger under the spring rim

Technique used in inserting the diaphragm

internal examination by the doctor will assess the correct size for each individual. The required size may change, particularly after a pregnancy as the vaginal tissues are stretched and a larger cap may be needed. The cap fits snugly into the vagina so that the cervix is completely covered with the membrane, preventing sperm deposited in the vagina from getting into the cervix. The woman is first taught how to feel her own cervix as she must be certain that when the diaphragm is correctly positioned the cervix is completely covered. This takes a little time and patience, but the skill is easily acquired and after a week most women will be confident enough to fit and remove the cap. Spermicidal jelly is usually smeared in the dome of the diaphragm and around the rim of the cap to give further protection.

It is usual to leave the diaphragm in place for about six hours after intercourse after which it is removed and washed. It may be left in the vagina for a longer period of time when further spermicidal jelly should be used. Apart from failure to protect against pregnancy – and the failure rate is very low – this method has virtually no complications, though some women

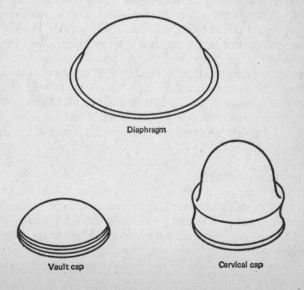

Diaphragm

Vault cap   Cervical cap

find the procedure of inserting, removing and washing the diaphragm irksome.

There are several other sorts of cap; one is shaped like a large thimble made of pink rubber and sits on the cervix by suction (cervical). Another type called a vault is a cross between this and the diaphragm. These are recommended when the neck of the womb is in an abnormal position or shorter than usual and the doctor will advise which type of diaphragm to use. The effectiveness of barrier methods preventing pregnancy is about 90 per cent.

The contraceptive Pill

In the early 1950s an American scientist, Gregory Pincus, first suggested that it might be possible to prevent a pregnancy with hormone tablets which effectively stop the egg being released by the ovary each month (ovulation). It had been known for some time that small doses of the female sex hormone, oestrogen, normally produced by the ovary in the first half of the menstrual cycle, could inhibit ovulation successfully but in the process almost always caused bleeding and irregular periods. It was also known that progesterone, which is a hormone produced in the second half of the menstrual cycle, was primarily concerned with keeping the menstrual cycle regular. For the next few years scientists concentrated on isolating a progesterone drug so that a suitable mixture of the two hormones could be taken in tablet form to prevent ovulation and maintain a normal menstrual pattern. The first contraceptive Pills were marketed in the early 1960s.

How do they work?
Although there are a host of different brands of contraceptive Pill available on the market today their mode of action is similar. In order for an egg to be formed and shed the ovary is stimulated by the pituitary gland in the brain which sends out special ripening messages or hormones. The Pill simply prevents the pituitary gland from putting out these ripening hormones and therefore ovulation will be suppressed.

How are they taken?

Every packet of contraceptive Pills has its own instruction leaflet and these should be followed precisely. Most Pills come in packages of twenty-one and the first tablet should be taken on the fifth day of menstruation (the first day of the period counts as day 1). One tablet a day should be taken, preferably at the same time of day, until the pack is finished; a gap of seven pill-free days follows, during which a period will occur. A new packet should be started after the seven pill-free days, regardless of whether a period has occurred or not. In this way a regular pattern will be established that is easy to remember and the schedule will be three weeks on the Pill and one week off. For those women who have difficulty in following this pattern a different brand of tablet is available which comes in a pack of twenty-eight. The first twenty-one Pills contain hormone and the last seven are dummies and one tablet is taken every day without a break.

Because the body takes a little time to react to these hormones the Pill may not be entirely successful in preventing ovulation during the first cycle and this is why it is safer to use additional forms of contraception during the first two weeks. If it becomes necessary to change the Pill similar precautions should be taken. Thereafter, if the Pill is taken as directed the success rate in preventing a pregnancy is virtually 100 per cent. Most women find that they are less liable to forget the Pill if it is taken first thing in the morning rather than at night. If the morning Pill is forgotten a Pill can be taken the same evening and this will not alter effectiveness in preventing conception. If the Pill is forgotten for two or more days bleeding may occur which can be ignored but additional methods of contraception should be used for the remainder of that cycle.

Side effects of the Pill

Some side effects are common during the first few weeks. Nausea and sickness, swollen and tender breasts, headaches, an increase in vaginal discharge, some weight gain or irregular spotting of blood are common. These complaints are usually temporary and often disappear after two or three cycles. If they do not settle the doctor should be consulted.

Apart from these minor effects there are certain long-term complications of oral contraception that must be considered. It is not uncommon for mood changes, particularly bouts of depression, to occur, and the desire for sex may be temporarily reduced. Sometimes an increase in sexual desire occurs, but rather than being directly due to the female hormone oestrogen this occurs mainly because the fear of pregnancy is removed and sex can take place without any worries or inhibitions.

The Pill may cause a small rise in the blood pressure and this is why blood pressure is measured every time the woman attends her doctor or family planning clinic. In fact blood pressure tends to increase with age and duration of Pill use and seems to be correlated with the dose of oestrogen. Sometimes switching brands of the Pill can eliminate this effect.

There is no proof whatsoever that the Pill causes cancer. The breast, however, is sensitive to the female sex hormone oestrogen and during the pre-menstrual phase of the cycle the breasts may feel lumpy and tender. If an unsuspected cancer of the breast exists the oestrogen content of the Pill can cause the growth to increase but in no way will it have caused the cancer to arise in the first place.

The Pill and future fertility
If a woman wishes to become pregnant the Pill should be stopped at the end of that packet. Often the periods may take a month or two to return, although this should cause no concern. It is ideal to wait for two or three periods before trying to get pregnant because the doctor will then be able to tell more accurately when the baby is due. This is because ovulation often occurs irregularly for a while after stopping the Pill and if the periods are also irregular calculations of the estimated date of delivery of a baby may be inaccurate.

Sometimes the periods take longer than two or three months to return and this may worry a woman who is trying to conceive. Though only 1 per cent of women who take the Pill do not menstruate once the Pill is discontinued, this complication can seldom be predicted. It seems, though, that those who have an irregular menstrual cycle or who missed periods frequently before going on the Pill are more prone to have trouble in this respect. Many doctors therefore do not recommend the Pill for women with very irregular menstruation. Most women on the Pill find that their periods are quite scanty and light and some may get no period at all. If no periods occur at the end of each 21-day cycle for three successive months the doctor should be informed. Provided the periods return after coming off the Pill there is no significance in absence of menstruation while taking it and the doctor may advise giving the Pill a break for a month or two to see whether the periods do return.

If the periods do not start and there is no wish for a pregnancy, no specific treatment is needed as menstruation almost always recurs within six months, and no harm at all is caused. If the couple wish to conceive, menstruation and ovulation can usually be induced with special tablets (Clomid) taken for five days every month (see Chapter 11). Occasionally periods do not return despite treatment with mild stimulating drugs. Should this occur tests may be needed to exclude other causes before sophisticated treatment with fertility drugs is tried. Though it is usually possible to get the periods restarted with treatment, a small number of women whose periods stop following the Pill remain resistant to fertility drugs and because menstruation and ovulation do not return their fertility may be impaired.

The most serious complication relating to the Pill is the possible occurrence of a blood clot in a vein (thrombosis). Although it is seldom possible to predict the likelihood of a thrombosis, recent research has indicated that the risks are higher in those over thirty-five who are overweight, smoke heavily and are taking a contraceptive Pill with a high dose of oestrogen.

To put the matter into perspective, the chance of a previously fit and healthy woman under the age of thirty-five developing a fatal thrombosis is less than 3 in 100,000 women, whereas the chances of this occurring in pregnancy are about twice as high because pregnancy predisposes to clotting of the blood. As well as this the death rate in women who had legal terminations of pregnancy in a quoted series was 7 per 100,000. The conclusion, therefore, is that staying on the Pill and avoiding pregnancy seems safer than being pregnant or having an abortion.

Medical research into the effects that the Pill has on the body, both immediate and long term, should eventually result in reducing the complications to a minimum. For the present there are still a number of questions about the Pill for which there are no definite answers. The press and advertising media may sometimes cause unnecessary anxiety for those on the Pill and discussion with friends and relatives can be more misleading than helpful.

Does the Pill have to be prescribed?
It has recently been suggested that the contraceptive Pill should be made available without a prescription and sold over the counter in any chemist, but there are good reasons why it is best to see a doctor first. The Pill could be inadvisable under certain circumstances, for example if there is evidence of a previous thrombosis in the leg, or if there is active disease that may interfere with Pill-taking such as diabetes. Examination by the doctor will ensure that no such conditions exist and that the genital organs are normal. Although each packet of contraceptive Pills contains a well-prepared leaflet outlining the way in which the Pill should be taken and what to do if there are problems it is helpful if these matters are explained by the doctor first.

How long is it safe to take the Pill?
Most doctors believe that although the Pill is not contra-indicated absolutely in the late thirties and early forties it is probably more sensible to seek alternative forms of birth control. Birth control Pills are potent hormones that affect many systems of the body; with advancing age natural changes do occur and it may be prudent to keep outside influences that may accelerate these changes to a minimum, particularly in the individual who is overweight and smokes heavily.

Is it necessary to come off the Pill for intervals to give the body a break?
Again advice may vary but there is no scientific evidence to suggest that discontinuation of the Pill for a few months makes any difference whatsoever to the frequency of complications or subsequent fertility, provided the periods occur regularly. If there

are no contra-indications, and no side effects develop, women may safely continue with the contraceptive Pill for as long as the doctor advises without a break.

If a pregnancy arises inadvertently while taking the Pill are there any dangers to the developing baby?

This question has been recently highlighted because it was found that certain tablets containing the same hormones as the Pill but in higher doses were used as a form of pregnancy test. These tablets used to be given for three or four days after a missed period and produced a small bleed if the woman was not pregnant. These drugs have recently been taken off the market, partly because there are more reliable methods of confirming pregnancy and also because it had been suggested that there was an increased incidence of abnormalities in the unborn children of women who had been given these tablets in the early weeks of pregnancy. However, there is no evidence to suggest that if a woman becomes pregnant while taking the contraceptive Pill similar effects may occur, though there is a slightly higher risk of miscarriage.

How soon can the Pill safely be restarted after pregnancy?

It is normal practice for a woman to wait for her first period before starting the Pill. If she is not breast feeding periods usually return within a few weeks of the birth of the baby. Breast-feeding mothers, however, often do not start their periods until lactation has finished and although it is extremely unlikely that a pregnancy will result in the absence of periods, it is possible. Commonly alternative methods of contraception are advised while breast feeding continues because the Pill can reduce the amount of milk produced by the breasts. Although some of the oestrogen content of the Pill can be transferred through the milk to the baby no harm will come to the infant. If menstruation does not recur after some months after breast feeding is discontinued there is no reason not to restart the Pill.

Can a period safely be postponed with the Pill?

If a period is going to coincide with an important event, say a holiday or crucial examination, bleeding can be prevented simply by continuing to take one Pill a day after the packet is finished without a break. As soon as it is convenient the Pill can be stopped and the next period should come within a few days. *Occasionally* changing the pattern of the periods in this way will cause no harm whatsoever but it is best to check with the doctor first.

Alternative contraceptive tablets

The contraceptive Pill that has been discussed consists of two hormones – oestrogen and progesterone – and it is the oestrogen hormone that is responsible for the side effects and complications; the progesterone hormone is virtually harmless. This fact has stimulated medical researchers to develop an effective method of contraception in tablet form that contains no oestrogen but progesterone alone. The first of such preparations was produced a few years ago and known as the 'Mini Pill'; this has now been superseded by vastly improved progesterone-only tablets which are becoming increasingly popular as an alternative to the contraceptive Pill.

These tablets work in a different way to the contraceptive Pill. Under normal circumstances the cervix liberates a fluid which attracts the sperm deposited during intercourse. The progesterone-only tablets change the consistency of this fluid so that the sperm are repelled from gaining entrance to the womb: in other words the discharge from the cervix becomes hostile to the sperm. If some sperm do get through the cervix the progesterone also makes it difficult for the egg to travel along the fallopian tube, partially prevents the sperm from penetrating the egg, and changes the consistency of the lining of the womb making it less receptive to the fertilized egg.

There are several different brands of progesterone-only tablets available on the market and they are all taken in the same way, that is, one tablet every morning without a break usually starting on day 1 of the period.

How effective are they?
Like any other form of contraception they are not quite as effec-

tive as the contraceptive Pill but the success rate is in the region of 95 per cent.

Are there any complications?

Although the progesterone-only Pills were developed mainly to avoid oestrogen-associated complications, some of the minor side effects seen with the combination Pill have been reported with the progesterone-only Pill – weight changes, vaginal discharge, occasional breast changes and minor mood variations may occur. The principal problem, however, concerns the periods themselves, whereas the combination Pill characteristically produces a short, regular period, the progesterone-only pill may cause irregular menstruation, heavy bleeding and sometimes absence of periods; though most women have no problems.

Originally suggested for use in breast-feeding mothers as a suitable alternative to other oral contraception as no inhibition of milk production occurs, the progesterone-only Pills are a satisfactory alternative method of contraception in those who cannot take the combination Pill or intra-uterine device but wish to use a tablet form of family planning.

The other alternative contraceptive Pill is the 'morning after' Pill. If tablets containing high doses of synthetic oestrogen are taken within three days of unprotected intercourse, implantation of the fertilized egg in the womb may be prevented. This method of family planning has little to recommend it as it is usually ineffective, can cause unpleasant side effects such as sickness, and possibly longer-term effects on the developing embryo.

The future of chemical contraception

Research work is in progress using injections of progesterone drugs every three to six months which work on similar principles. This method is already in use in some underdeveloped countries but is still at the research stage in the United Kingdom. Hormone tablets which temporarily reduce the production and effectiveness of sperm in the male have been used on volunteers but have not proved effective.

The intra-uterine device (IUD or coil)

Centuries ago camel drivers in the Middle East recognized that pebbles placed in the uterus of the animal prevented pregnancies during long trips in the desert. This principle led to the knowledge that any foreign body inside the human uterus will act in the same way. The materials originally used were metals consisting of gold, platinum or silver, but because these caused unpleasant reactions in the uterus they have now been entirely replaced by special forms of plastic causing little or no reaction in the uterus.

Modern IUDs come in different shapes and sizes, easily regain their shape after insertion into the uterus and end in a thread or tail which hangs for 2 cm outside the cervix so that their presence can be confirmed.

How do they work?

The precise mode of action is uncertain but it is believed that the presence of a foreign body in the womb sets up a minor degree of inflammation in its walls, preventing the fertilized egg from implantation. There is little evidence to support the belief that the IUD causes the uterus to expel the fertilized egg as in a miscarriage.

Some of the latest IUDs have certain metal or hormones incorporated in the device in minute amounts which increase the effectiveness of preventing a pregnancy by altering the chemical composition of the lining cells of the womb and making the environment unsuitable for the fertilized egg.

The effectiveness of an IUD preventing a pregnancy is second only to the combined oral contraceptive Pill and has the great advantage of convenience. Once inserted contraceptive worries are over and there is no need to use additional creams, foams or jellies. As the device is inserted by a doctor and there is no need for either partner to take an active role in contraception this method has proved extremely effective in underdeveloped countries. Before the newer smaller types of IUD were produced intra-uterine contraception was limited to those who had already had children because it was easier to insert the IUD

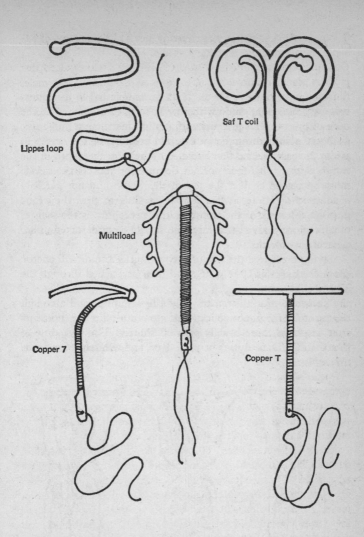

Lippes loop

Saf T coil

Multiload

Copper 7

Copper T

Intra-uterine devices

through a cervix which had already been stretched by child-birth. This limitation is no longer valid.

How is insertion done?

It is common practice for an IUD to be inserted in a doctor's surgery or hospital clinic without any form of anaesthetic. The neck of the womb is grasped with a blunt instrument and a fine probe is passed through the external opening of the cervix to assess the ease of insertion and also to measure the depth of the womb cavity. This is important because for success the device must be placed against the top of the womb and not partially inside it. Sometimes, when it is impossible to pass the probe through the neck of the womb or this procedure is too painful the doctor may advise that insertion should be undertaken under general anaesthetic.

Having measured the size of the womb the doctor will choose the correct size of IUD which will then be pushed through the neck of the womb.

The whole procedure takes only a few minutes and although it is common for minor colicky pains to occur for a few moments after insertion these usually pass off shortly. The best time to insert an IUD is during a period or immediately afterwards

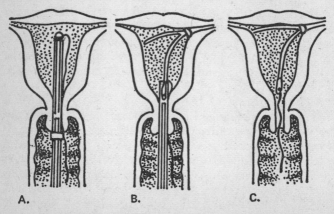

A.   B.   C.

The insertion of a copper 7

because the cervix is soft and stretchable at this time and there can be no possibility of the woman being pregnant.

After a pregnancy it is usual to wait until the post-natal visit some six weeks after delivery before considering an IUD because by this time the womb will have returned to its normal size and there will be less chance of rejection. An IUD can be inserted immediately after termination of a pregnancy though the chance of rejection is slightly higher than normal.

Removal of an IUD is simple; the doctor will merely pull on the tail or thread; this procedure is usually painless and takes a few seconds only.

What are the side effects?
Pain and bleeding may continue after insertion for a few days or even weeks, though this is unusual. The pain is usually due to the womb contracting – similar to labour – because it recognizes that a foreign body is present. Perseverance is worthwhile because these symptoms usually disappear after the first period. The bleeding pattern of menstruation is often altered and it is not unusual for periods to become heavier and perhaps irregular. Again these symptoms often settle after the first two or three months. Women are generally taught how to locate the thread of the IUD so that a check may be made at regular intervals, preferably just after a period, to ensure that the IUD has not come out, or to see the doctor within a few weeks after insertion and thereafter at three, six or twelve monthly intervals. Expulsion of an IUD does not necessarily imply complete failure of that method and it is generally possible for a further insertion to be attempted, perhaps with a different type of IUD.

A lost thread may not mean that the IUD has been expelled. Commonly the string gets pulled up through the neck of the womb so that it lies curled up in the body of the womb. If this is suspected then a scan test or X-ray is usually taken to confirm that the IUD is still present and if it is, there is no need for its immediate removal. The IUD with a lost thread may eventually have to be removed under general anaesthesia because there is no string to pull and the neck of the womb may have to be stretched.

Infection of the womb and the fallopian tubes does occasionally occur but the incidence has been greatly reduced by modern sterile techniques during insertion as well as the use of less irritant forms of IUD.

The failure rate with an IUD is about 3 per cent. If pregnancy occurs with an IUD in place there is a small chance of a miscarriage in the first few weeks, but there is no evidence to suggest that the developing baby is affected in any other way should the pregnancy proceed. Medical opinion varies as to the best course of treatment if this complication occurs. Formerly no attempt at removal of the IUD was made and it was usually recovered after the birth of the baby, often lodged in the placenta or afterbirth. Because there have been recent reports of serious infection occuring during pregnancy with some forms of IUD there are those who believe that the IUD should be removed if possible by gently pulling on the string as soon as a pregnancy has been confirmed. Removal of a coil during pregnancy usually causes no problems and suggestions that a baby will be born abnormal or deformed should a pregnancy continue with an IUD in the uterus are totally without foundation.

Sometimes the thread that lies outside the cervix irritates the partner's penis and intercourse may become painful for him. This is usually because the thread is too short rather than too long and the doctor will usually be able to adjust things accordingly.

Finally there is no evidence to suggest that any form of IUD causes a cancer to develop in the neck or the body of the womb.

An IUD is inadvisable in women who suffer from heavy and painful periods, who have suffered infection in the pelvis, or if large fibroids are present in the uterus. Certain general diseases may also prohibit the use of an IUD and the doctor is the best person to advise about this.

Other contraceptive techniques

Foams, jellies and certain chemicals are easily available in chemist shops, are cheap and easy to use but are only 80 per cent effective in preventing a pregnancy. They are inserted into the vagina before intercourse by means of an applicator and usually

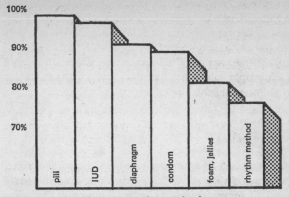

100% ─

90% ─

80% ─

70% ─

pill

IUD

diaphragm

condom

foam, jellies

rhythm method

Effectiveness of contraceptive methods.
The probability of avoiding pregnancy on the basis of past usage

act by killing the sperm on contact; they must be reapplied into the vagina after a single act of intercourse as effectiveness is only temporary.

Some women like to douche the vagina after intercourse but this technique has little to recommend it as a form of contraception as it is unreliable.

About 90,000 women in this country are pregnant before marriage and 120,000 women undergo legal termination of pregnancy every year. Despite the increased availability of free contraception there remains a great need for advertising this fact and educating people in the principles of family planning. It is important for those who do seek advice to understand one basic principle: most of the side effects and complications of any form of contraception are relative and the correct contraceptive must be tailored to the individual's needs. For example a woman in the 'at risk' age group of oral contraception, i.e. in late thirties who smokes heavily, may still want to take the small risk of problems with the Pill if no other method of contraception is suitable and 100 per cent protection from pregnancy is necessary. Similarly, the woman who has heavy periods may prefer to run the risk of increasing this problem with the intra-uterine device rather than be forced to change her method of family planning to the contraceptive Pill with its own special complications.

At present there is no perfect method of contraception which would give 100 per cent efficiency, be cheap and easy to take, be instantly reversible, require little motivation and have no side effects. Each couple guided by their doctor must make a choice of the method that suits them best at any particular time.

Sterilization

Sterilization is an unfortunate word because although it is taken to mean a procedure for rendering a man or woman incapable of producing offspring the implication may wrongfully be taken to imply an alteration in sexual feelings and performance. It is the most effective and the most final form of birth control and should be considered to all intents and purposes irreversible. Sterilization procedures usually involve the surgical interruption of the fallopian tubes in the female and the vas deferens, which is a tube leading from the testes or sperm sac to the penis, in the male.

Female sterilization

There are many different techniques of blocking off the fallopian tubes. They can be divided, tied, burnt (cauterized) or removed and each surgeon will have his preferred method. There are also two methods of approach; either a special torch (laparoscope – see Chapter 14) is inserted into the abdomen just underneath the navel, and by means of an instrument which can be passed down the sheath of the torch the fallopian tube can be grasped and burnt or closed with a ring or clip; or the abdomen is opened by a full cut and the tubes are divided or removed.

The torch (laparoscope) method
This method has the great advantage of speed and economy. Though occasionally performed under local anaesthetic, in the

great majority of instances a full anaesthetic is used and admission to hospital for one or two nights is necessary. Because the procedure is performed through one or two minute cuts in the abdomen which only require one stitch into the skin the woman can be home within forty-eight hours. The success rate of this procedure is around 99 per cent. The occasional pregnancy that occurs after this operation is due either to an unsuspected pregnancy being already present before operation (though this can be avoided by choosing the correct time in the menstrual cycle to do the operation, ideally just after a period) or, rarely, because the two ends of the tube that have been destroyed by burning, or occluded by a clip or ring, join up again. Apart from these the only other disadvantage of the procedure is that in some instances the menstrual flow may tend to become heavier.

Tying or removal of tubes

Although by no means major surgery this procedure does involve a formal cut into the abdomen so that the tubes may actually be tied or removed and this will inevitably involve the patient in a longer stay in hospital with the discomfort of an abdominal scar – though it is usually only 5 to 8 cm in length and placed in the pubic hairline so that once healed it is invisible. This method is preferred by some surgeons because the success rate is virtually 100 per cent (though even with this method pregnancies have resulted) or when laparoscopy is unsuitable (see Chapter 14).

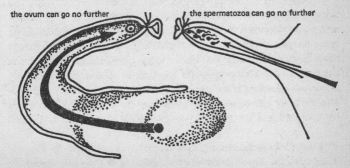

the ovum can go no further   the spermatozoa can go no further

Result of division of the fallopian tubes

It is also the method of choice if sterilization is performed immediately after childbirth or during Caesarian section. Sterilization operations involving interruption of the fallopian tubes cause no alteration in the egg production mechanism of the ovaries and the egg simply becomes absorbed. Neither is there any hormone change or physical alteration in the way in which the reproductive organs work. It is simply a procedure that causes a mechanical barrier to the passage of the egg in the tube.

Sterilization by removal of the womb (hysterectomy) has a small but definite indication. It is usually reserved for the woman over forty with existing trouble such as excessively heavy periods, fibroids or a very early growth in the womb. In this instance it would seem illogical to perform a short quick operation with the laparoscope only to find that hysterectomy might become necessary anyway in a year or two's time.

Some surgeons may advise hysterectomy in the older woman in the absence of disease in the womb as it is argued that if no further children are desired the uterus becomes a useless organ and with advancing age is more prone to be the seat of menstrual problems and cancer. Against this argument, hysterectomy has more risks than the smaller operations, is a major procedure, and may have psychological repercussions.

Newer methods of female sterilization
Operations on the fallopian tube can be performed through the vagina under certain circumstances but this operation is not commonly done in the United Kingdom. Advantages include no post-operative discomfort, no visible scar and early discharge from hospital. Because this operation is done entirely through the vagina the operating space is more limited and the technique not always easy. It is not usually advised immediately after childbirth because the fallopian tubes may be inaccessible from the vaginal end and the vaginal tissues are very congested and bleed easily.

Two new techniques are currently being used for female sterilization. One involves the passing of a telescope-like instrument through the vagina and into the neck of the womb so that the internal openings of the fallopian tubes into the womb can be identified and blocked either by a hot current or certain chemicals. This instrument is called a hysteroscope which can also be used in order to examine the inside of the womb in certain gynaecological conditions. The other method employs the use of a laser beam applied externally to the fallopian tubes. This technique has not yet been perfected but laser beams are already being used successfully for the treatment of a number of medical conditions.

Male sterilization (vasectomy)

This is the male equivalent of tubal tying. It consists of dividing the tube along which the sperm are transported from the testes to the penis called a vas deferens. Because each vas is situated just under the skin on either side of the scrotal sac, locating and dividing this channel is a much easier procedure than any form of female sterilization. Moreover, it is often done under local anaesthetic in the outpatient department. A small cut is made into the top end of the scrotal sac, the vas is found and a small section cut out with the remaining ends tied off. The wound is closed with a few stitches and the whole procedure takes only about twenty minutes. There is usually a little discomfort and swelling of the scrotal sac for the first few days. Unlike female sterilization it is necessary to use alternative methods of birth control until the doctor advises that this is no longer necessary. This will be judged by the examination of at least two semen specimens over a two-month period to confirm complete absence of sperms. Each surgeon will have his own routine for follow-up which should be strictly adhered to for maximum efficiency. Contrary to the myths surrounding this operation vasectomy leaves the male genital system unchanged. There is no alteration in the output of male hormones or the ability to perform sexually. Erection and ejaculation occur in the same way as before and there is no change in the amount of semen produced, although of course no sperm is present.

*

Though most sterilization procedures have a virtual 100 per cent success rate, their efficiency as birth control measured in social terms depends largely on the initial interview and counselling by the doctor. Attitudes in lay and medical circles have changed dramatically in the past ten years. It used to be normal for the procedure to be reserved for a woman over the age of thirty-five who had at least three or four children and could not get on with any of the recognized forms of contraception. It is now quite usual for sterilization requests to be made by women at any age for personal reasons.

Is male or female sterilization reversible?

If only a small section of fallopian tube in the female or vas deferens in the male is occluded it should in theory be possible to rejoin the normal portions of the remaining tubes and restore fertility. For the present time, however, the overall results of this procedure are disappointing. This is largely because the fallopian tube and the vas deferens are made up of extremely delicate tissue and although the actual technique of rejoining these tubes is not difficult they tend to block up again soon after surgery. Even if reconnection of the vas in the male is successful there is a marked reduction in the efficiency of the remaining sperm because of the presence of so-called antibodies which are produced by the male in response to the vasectomy operation. For these reasons doctors usually advise the couple that any sterilization procedure should be regarded as an irrevocable step.

If a woman who has been sterilized wishes to conceive, the feasibility of reversal would depend largely on which method of sterilization was used. If the tubes were simply occluded by a clip using the laparoscope or torch it is possible to remove the clip but the crushed section of the tube will normally have to be removed and the ends joined. Burning the tubes causes considerable damage to the tube lining and restoration of normal activity is more difficult. If the tubes have been removed then, of course, the position is hopeless. Transplanting a fallopian tube removed from another woman or inserting a graft in place of the absent tube have not met with success. If all fails then the woman's only chance of conception is by fertilization outside the body (see Chapter 11).

The success rate in reversing sterilization procedures in men is higher than in women, though the often quoted figure of 25 per cent is probably unrealistic.

A well-motivated couple who understand the principles involved in sterilization will be happy with the result; those who have been coerced into asking for sterilization or who harbour fears that the procedure will involve an alteration in femininity and sexual feelings may suffer from psychological upsets largely as a result of guilt.

Points to note

1 Advice about family planning is freely available to women of all ages in the United Kingdom and there is a wide choice of contraceptives. Go and talk to your family doctor or your local family planning clinic if you want help.

2 The contraceptive Pill is the most efficient method of birth control. It is virtually 100 per cent reliable in preventing a pregnancy if taken as directed.

3 There is no evidence to indicate that the Pill causes cancer.

4 The small risk of thrombosis due to the Pill is increased if you are over thirty-five, overweight and smoke heavily.

5 Do not be surprised if your periods take a month or two to return after you come off the Pill.

6 Although it is best to wait for two normal periods before planning to have a baby, if you should accidentally get pregnant while on the Pill, it is highly unlikely that any harm will come to the developing baby.

7 Remember to use additional birth control
   (a) if you forget to take the Pill for more than two days
   (b) for a fortnight when you first start the Pill
   (c) if you have been sick or had diarrhoea for a few days
   (d) if you change from one Pill to another.

8 Though not quite as reliable as the Pill, intra-uterine devices provide extremely effective birth control.

9 If you have had a pregnancy, and your periods are not naturally heavy, modern IUDs cause few problems and will not cause a deformity in a developing baby should an accidental pregnancy occur.

10 Sterilization procedures in men and women simply block the
tubes conveying the sperm or eggs. No untoward changes
occur in the body and rather than reducing sexual desire and
performance the reverse is often true as intercourse can take
place freely without fear of an unwanted pregnancy.

9 Premature interruption of pregnancy

Abortion and miscarriage describe exactly the same thing, i.e. the interruption or loss of a pregnancy before the end of the 28th week regardless of whether the abortion occurs by chance or is induced deliberately. In British law a baby born after the 28th week of pregnancy is considered to be viable or capable of surviving and therefore pregnancies cannot be terminated after this time, though the chances of a baby surviving at this early stage of pregnancy are remote.

The great majority of abortions occur spontaneously and these will be discussed first.

Spontaneous abortion (miscarriage)

This complication of pregnancy is extremely common. Between 15 and 20 per cent of all pregnancies will end in miscarriage and often for no obvious reason. A spontaneous miscarriage is more likely to occur if the mother suffers from a general medical disease such as diabetes, heart and kidney disorders, or abnormalities of the pelvic organs such as fibroids or a double uterus, but commonly no cause is found. There may be something wrong with the chromosome or make-up cells of the baby in the first few weeks of pregnancy, resulting in some structural abnormality. Because nature tends to discard what is not normal the human uterus is more likely to expel its contents and a miscarriage will occur. Unfortunately this is not always the case as not all deformities are incompatible with life.

Although incidental occurrences that happen in the first few weeks of pregnancy are often blamed for causing a miscarriage – minor accidents, overwork, mental strain, excessive exercise, travel, stomach upsets and so on – the embryo that is destined to stay inside the uterus clings very strongly to its new bed, a fact borne out by failure of women to procure an abortion themselves by taking various medicines and drugs.

One well-recognized cause of miscarriage called incompetence of the cervix encourages expulsion of the products of the womb at a later stage in pregnancy, usually between eighteen and twenty-four weeks. This occurs because the neck of the cervix may be wider than usual, with the result that the contents of the womb tend to slide through the open cervix and be expelled.

What are the signs of a miscarriage?

The first sign of a threatening miscarriage is bleeding from the vagina which usually occurs after the first or second missed period. If the bleeding is slight and there is no pain the prognosis for the outcome of pregnancy is good and in most instances the bleeding will stop and the pregnancy will proceed normally. If the bleeding becomes heavier accompanied by cramp-like pains the chances of the pregnancy proceeding are less good. Any bleeding that occurs in pregnancy should be reported to the doctor; he will probably do an internal examination which will help to decide whether the miscarriage is still at the threatening stage or is becoming inevitable. Contrary to popular belief, gentle internal examination does not cause or promote a miscarriage.

If the cervix is tightly shut as it is in the non-pregnant state, the bleeding may stop and all may be well; if the neck of the womb is starting to stretch and open as it would in labour then it is more likely that a miscarriage has become inevitable. It is not always easy to differentiate between these two stages and this is why women are often admitted to hospital for observation, bed-rest and further investigation. Usually nature declares its intention within a few days and either the bleeding stops and the pregnancy continues, or bleeding continues with pain, and miscarriage will occur.

The usual treatment for the woman who is threatening to

miscarry is rest either at home or in hospital, and avoidance of sexual intercourse until the bleeding has stopped. As it would be impossible to admit every woman in the early stages of pregnancy to hospital, admission is usually reserved for those in whom the pregnancy is particularly precious, such as a pregnancy occurring for the first time in the older woman, or when previous miscarriages have occurred. Sometimes hormone injections are given when the pregnancy is threatening to miscarry to help the embryo anchor itself firmly to the wall of the womb, but apart from rest there is no other specific treatment that will influence the outcome of a threatened miscarriage. If the bleeding stops and the pregnancy continues the woman may be reassured that no harm has come to the developing baby and it has the same chance of being born normal as if no bleeding had occurred.

If the miscarriage progresses and bleeding continues the uterus will start to contract, causing pain, and admission to hospital is necessary as bleeding can become quite heavy and will only stop when the uterus has been emptied spontaneously or by a small operation known as a D & C (see Chapter 14).

Sometimes fragments of tissue are passed mixed with blood and this usually indicates that the abortion is *incomplete*. This is potentially the most dangerous form of miscarriage because severe bleeding may occur quite suddenly if any of the contents of the womb have not been expelled. Treatment consists again of admission to hospital and surgical evacuation of the womb.

Missed abortion

Occasionally the woman may notice that the feelings of pregnancy that were present in the early weeks, such as tingling of the breasts and nausea, may subside, or she may just 'not feel pregnant any more', and the doctor may find at a routine antenatal visit that the womb has not grown in size since the last attendance. Here there are no outward signs to the patient that anything is wrong and no bleeding occurs, but the baby may have died inside the womb. If this diagnosis is suspected there is no need for any immediate active management. It could be that the baby is merely resting and continued observation over the next few weeks will confirm whether the womb is getting larger or not. There is no need for anxiety if a conservative policy is adopted because no harm will come to the mother even if the baby is dead and retained within the womb, and it may not be advisable for any immediate interference. Normally the diagnosis is confirmed by ultrasound scan tests, urinary pregnancy tests and repeated observation of the size of the uterus by the doctor, and if there is convincing evidence that the baby is dead the woman will probably be admitted to hospital so that the uterus can be emptied by scraping the womb.

Once the miscarriage is over and the womb is empty the body adjusts itself quickly to the normal non-pregnant state and periods will start again, usually within a few weeks. If the couple wish to try for another pregnancy soon there is no need to wait longer than two or three months, though it is better to have at least two periods before starting to conceive again, because if a pregnancy occurs sooner it is often difficult to know when conception took place and hence to calculate when the baby should be due. Advice should always be sought from the doctor before embarking on a subsequent pregnancy.

Recurrent miscarriage

Unfortunately some women have a tendency to suffer repeated miscarriages. Sometimes a cause can be found after careful blood and urine tests, X-rays of the womb and chromosome studies. Known causes include medical diseases such as untreated diabetes, thyroid disorders, certain infectious diseases, abnormalities of the womb such as large fibroids, an incompetent cervix (see Chapter 11), or the woman may have a defective chromosome structure which may be diagnosed by special blood tests. Some of these abnormalities may be treated successfully but for others, such as chromosome defects, there is no cure.

If no cause is found the management of a subsequent pregnancy will depend largely on the views of the individual gynaecologist. Commonly admission for bed-rest in hospital is advised as soon as pregnancy has been confirmed. Hormone injections to help stabilize the growing embryo may be given together with iron and vitamin tablets, but the mainstay of treatment is purely rest. No one really understands why bed-rest improves chances of success except that it is known that inactivity improves the flow of blood and oxygen to the afterbirth or placenta, encouraging growth of the baby. Bed-rest may be advised for as long as three to four months, or at least two weeks later than the time at which the previous miscarriage occurred. It is surprising how often this simple régime is successful.

Induced abortion

Inducing an abortion is the oldest known method of population control. For centuries it was widely practised and tolerated in many societies in the world. Following the declaration by Pope Pius IX in the 1860s that all abortions were murder, laws were passed in most Western countries outlawing abortion unless it was necessary to save the woman's life. It was not for 100 years, until 1967, that a new abortion act became law in the UK legalizing abortion under certain well-defined circumstances. Though by no means supported by all, the change towards liberal attitudes with abortions has occurred partly for cultural reasons and partly because so many women suffered irreparable harm and occasionally death following self-induced abortions or when abortions were procured illegally.

Abortion today is illegal in certain countries, notably those with a predominantly Roman Catholic faith such as France, Spain and Italy; legal, under certain circumstances, in Britain and the USA; and obtainable on demand in some countries such as Hungary and Japan.

British law allows the legal termination of pregnancy before 28 weeks if two independent medical practitioners agree that the continuation of the pregnancy would involve greater risk to the life, physical or mental health of the mother or her existing children than if the pregnancy were terminated.

A pregnancy can also be terminated if there is a substantial risk that the unborn child would be born with a serious mental or physical deformity. Unfortunately, the likelihood of congenital abnormality cannot always be predicted but there are certain conditions that can now be diagnosed with great accuracy in the early months of pregnancy.

The chances of a mongol child being born to healthy parents increases with maternal age. It is comparatively rare under the age of thirty but over forty the incidence is around one in seventy This condition can be accurately diagnosed by withdrawing a sample of fluid surrounding the baby through a needle inserted into the mother's uterus (amniocentesis) and examining the specimen of fluid for the characteristic pattern of abnormal chromosome make-up that is known to exist in a mongol child.

Certain diseases affecting the spinal cord and the brain of the unborn child (spina bifida and hydrocephalus) may also be diagnosed with reasonable accuracy by blood and fluid tests. Because the number of laboratories in the UK with the expert equipment and staff to examine the fluid for these abnormalities is limited, each laboratory will have its own minimum maternal age limit which it will accept. If the mother has had no previous abnormal children most laboratories will only agree to test women aged thirty-eight and over. If, however, there is a history of a mongol child or a child with spina bifida, testing is usually available in a subsequent pregnancy.

There are other important aspects to consider regarding pre-natal diagnosis of disease. Amniocentesis cannot be done until the fourth month of pregnancy because before this time the cells of the fluid are not mature enough. Also, because of the nature of the laboratory tests results may not be available for a few weeks, by which time the pregnancy may be reasonably advanced. If an abnormality is confirmed termination of pregnancy will then have to be carried out by means other than simple evacuation of the uterus (see later this chapter). Perhaps by this time the mother has felt her baby moving and may feel a close affinity to her unborn child and the prospect of termination of pregnancy may become less acceptable even if an abnormality is likely. Though withdrawing fluid from the sac surrounding the baby is a simple, quick procedure taking only a few minutes and causing no more discomfort than a pinprick there is a small but definite incidence of miscarriage (1 per cent) and all these considerations need to be discussed carefully before the test is done.

The other common indication for terminating a pregnancy in the early weeks concerns the likelihood of abnormalities caused by the German measles virus. If a pregnant woman has contracted German measles (rubella) within the first twelve weeks of pregnancy or has come into contact with another infected person blood tests can show whether the virus of German measles has recently passed through the mother's blood to affect her baby. If infection in the unborn child occurs in the first eight weeks of pregnancy there is a substantial risk that the baby will be born with certain abnormalities. After ten weeks the risks diminish and after twelve weeks the risks of problems are small. There are a number of different abnormalties that can affect the baby including deafness, blindness and heart diseases. It is now routine practice for pregnant women attending for their first visit to have a blood test which determines whether they have contracted German measles in the past as this will almost certainly guarantee protection from any future infection. An injection of German measles vaccine is given to the non-immune mother after the birth of the baby. In many parts of the country this vaccine is being offered to schoolgirls and teenagers as part of a screening programme. It is obviously important to use adequate contraception for at least two months after the vaccine is given.

As previously mentioned, in this country the decision legalizing termination of pregnancy must be made by two medical practitioners and they are required by law to sign a form to this effect. A woman requesting an abortion is normally referred by her general practitioner to a gynaecologist or to one of the registered charitable organizations that carry out terminations of pregnancy. Because this system of referral often takes time and because termination of a pregnancy after twelve weeks becomes a more complicated procedure it is important that the woman with an unwanted pregnancy consult her doctor as soon as possible.

How is termination of pregnancy performed ?
Provided the baby is small enough, and this usually corresponds to a pregnancy not more than twelve to fourteen weeks from the first day of the last normal period, the uterus is emptied through

a small flexible plastic tube passed through the neck of the womb connected to a suction apparatus. The earlier the pregnancy the more simple the procedure and ideally this operation should be performed by the eighth week of pregnancy. Between eight and twelve weeks this method of termination is still perfectly satisfactory but becomes slightly more difficult. Usually termination is done under general anaesthesia requiring a stay in hospital for one or two nights. In a few centres the operation is performed under local anaesthetic up to eight weeks of pregnancy. Commonly there is a little bleeding for a few days after termination. Discomfort is usually minimal though there may be cramp-like abdominal pains for the first day or so. There is no set time for the periods to return afterwards but menstruation usually recommences after a few weeks and the first two periods may be irregular and heavier than normal. Should bleeding continue for longer than a few days, or become heavy with abdominal pain, the doctor should be notified.

After twelve to fourteen weeks the foetus is too large to be removed through the neck of the womb and termination of pregnancy is carried out by one of two different methods. One involves a surgical operation carried out through the abdomen, similar to a Caesarian section operation. This method of terminating a pregnancy is not commonly performed because of possible future complications resulting from a scar in the uterus. It has been replaced by the administration of certain drugs which cause the womb to contract as in labour so that eventually the pregnancy miscarries. The substance used is derived from a series of drugs called Prostaglandins which are given either by direct injections into the womb or by instillation through the neck of the womb. Whichever method is used these drugs cause the uterus to contract so that the woman will have to undergo a mini-labour which may take a number of hours before miscarriage is complete. Once over it is often necessary to perform a D & C to ensure that the womb is completely empty.

Complications of termination of pregnancy
The earlier the pregnancy the fewer the complications of termination and the risks of the procedure up to ten weeks are negligible.

Fortunately nowadays serious infection is rare following legal abortion. Before the Abortion Act was introduced in the UK in 1967 desperation led many women with unwanted pregnancies to the back streets and the abortionist parlours. Attempts at producing abortions were made usually by unqualified personnel using unsterile instruments with the result that infection was introduced into the womb with catastrophic consequences and even sometimes death of the unfortunate woman.

It is significant that the number of septic abortions since 1967 has been dramatically reduced and this serious complication is now extremely rare. However, even if termination of pregnancy is properly carried out in an operating theatre with sterile instruments infection can occur, and although it is extremely uncommon for any serious impairment of the woman's health, mild infection in the womb may spread to the fallopian tubes, occasionally resulting in tubal blockage.

Incompetency of the cervix (see Chapter 11) may arise following termination especially if the pregnancy is over twelve weeks as the cervix necessarily has to be stretched in order to allow the instrument to be passed through. This complication may cause a miscarriage in a subsequent pregnancy.

To most women the end of an unplanned pregnancy is an enormous relief. Some, however, may develop psychological problems, perhaps due to guilt, and with the passage of time attitudes about the pregnancy may change. One estimate based on a large series of women whose pregnancies were terminated in Sweden suggested that 25 per cent of women suffered some sort of psychological upset in later life. The ultimate decision as to whether a pregnancy should be terminated must be made by the woman and her medical advisors. Health visitors and medical social workers may give considerable help through their knowledge of any relevant social circumstances as well as outlining help that may be available to the woman who has decided to keep her pregnancy. There is good evidence to show that the incidence of psychiatric problems that occur following termination can be greatly reduced by skilful and sympathetic counselling beforehand.

Ectopic pregnancy

The word 'ectopic' means misplaced, and an ectopic pregnancy is one that grows somewhere other than its normal site –namely the uterus; but for all intents and purposes the only place that a pregnancy can grow other than the uterus is the fallopian tube itself where fertilization of the egg by the male sperm takes place. Exceedingly rarely a pregnancy could form in the ovary and cases have been reported in the medical literature of a pregnancy actually growing to a fairly advanced stage free in the abdomen.

However, when doctors talk about ectopic pregnancy this is usually synonymous with a pregnancy in the fallopian tube.

How does this occur?

Three or four days after fertilization has taken place in the fallopian tube the fertilized egg passes down the tube towards the uterus where it sinks into the prepared bed in the lining of the uterus to start its growth as an embryo. Although the distance between the tube and the uterus is not great the journey of the fertilized egg can be quite perilous and migration along the tube can only occur if the tube is absolutely healthy, and the hairs inside the lining waft the fertilized egg along, and provided there is no obstruction or blockage to its passage. When an obstruction occurs in the tube preventing the fertilized egg from reaching the uterus the three-day-old pregnancy will start to grow in the tube itself.

Often no particular cause for the obstruction is found or the lining of the tube may not have developed normally. Sometimes the tube can be damaged by previous infection or the canal merely kinked as a result of previous surgery in the abdomen.

Basically, such a pregnancy is doomed to failure because as the pregnancy grows it distends the outer wall of the tube which is only relatively thin compared to the thick spongy muscle bed of the uterus where a pregnancy should normally grow. This stretching of the tube by the pregnancy will cause a lower abdominal pain on the affected side together with a little bleeding from the vagina. Untreated, the pregnancy will eventually burst through the tube causing acute pain and internal bleeding and sometimes the woman's collapse. For this reason it is extremely important to report one-sided abdominal pain or any vaginal bleeding that occurs in the very early weeks of a pregnancy.

What is the treatment?

If an ectopic pregnancy is suspected the diagnosis must be confirmed by surgical exploration or laparoscopy. Unfortunately, removing the pregnancy from the tube and reconstituting the tube lining is seldom satisfactory as the risk of a further tubal pregnancy at a later stage is increased by operating on the tube. The usual treatment, therefore, is to remove the whole tube with the tubal pregnancy in it, provided of course the tube on the other side has first been inspected and found to be normal. Although usually the pregnancy arises in the middle of the tube occasionally it may migrate towards the outer end and can be milked through the tube but this is very much the exception.

Provided one healthy tube remains there is little alteration to future fertility and the majority of women who have had one tube removed are able to conceive and have a normal pregnancy. A second ectopic pregnancy occurring in the remaining tube is extremely rare.

Points to note

1 The words miscarriage and abortion mean exactly the same thing, i.e. the loss of a pregnancy before the 28th week – pregnancy usually lasting for 40 weeks.
2 Spontaneous miscarriage is common; perhaps 20 per cent of all pregnancies ending in this way.
3 Though there are some well-recognized causes, miscarriage often occurs for no known reason and usually in the very early weeks.
4 Slight bleeding in the early pregnancy does not necessarily imply that a miscarriage will occur but you should inform your doctor.
5 If the bleeding stops there is no reason why the pregnancy should not continue normally, nor is there any increased

likelihood that the baby will be born deformed.

6 If you do miscarry, do not blame yourself. It is unlikely that you will have influenced the outcome of the pregnancy by overwork or stress.

7 Your periods should return within a few weeks of a miscarriage and there is actually no need to wait longer than two or three months before trying again but discuss this with your doctor first.

8 If you need help about an unwanted pregnancy go and chat to your doctor as soon as possible. Delay in seeking advice may prejudice the outcome, and the complications of termination of pregnancy increase with advancing weeks.

9 Persistent pain in the abdomen in the first few weeks of a pregnancy should be reported to your doctor. This is one of the symptoms of a pregnancy in the fallopian tube.

10 If one tube has to be removed because of an ectopic pregnancy and the remaining tube is normal, there is no reason why you should not have a normal pregnancy next time.

10 Sexual activity

Normal sexual activity

Sexual intercourse or coitus means that the male sex organ is placed in the body of the female partner. Although a woman's response to love-making depends on many factors including her age, general health, education, mood and intensity of foreplay, there are four recognized phases in the process of the sexual act.

The first phase is called the *excitement phase* and is concerned with sexual arousal, usually initiated by kissing and bodily contact. The excitement stage takes much longer to initiate in the woman than the man. The response to the initial arousal may be accentuated by visual attraction to the partner and seems to be related to certain times in the menstrual cycle. It is often said that women have a higher sexual interest just before or even during menstruation.

During the excitement phase certain changes occur in the breasts and in the genital organs. The nipples become swollen and erect and the breasts may noticeably increase in size. The outer lips of the vulva stretch upwards and outwards exposing the vaginal entrance in readiness for the penis to be inserted, and the vaginal walls become moist and lubricated as fluid is exuded from the glands inside the vagina. The heart rate rises and the blood pressure increases and the woman may be aware of her heart pounding pleasurably against the chest wall.

As stimulation of the genital organs continues the excitement phase heightens and the woman is ready for the erect penis to be inserted into the vagina. The lower end of the vagina actually becomes slightly narrower so that the penis can be gripped firmly. This is called the *plateau phase*.

The continued thrusting movements of the penis against the clitoris eventually produce the climax or *orgasm* and the muscles of the womb and the vagina contract forcibly giving rise to the gratifying tension-releasing jerking movements as climax is reached.

When orgasm is over the *resolution phase* begins. For half an hour or more after orgasm, if love-making does not continue, the swelling of the genital organs decreases and all the muscles relax, so the uterus, the vagina, the lips and the clitoris gradually return to the pre-arousal state. Immediately after climax the clitoris is extremely sensitive but this fades after a few seconds though the uterus, which may have become twice as big as normal during love-making, may take up to half an hour to return to its normal size.

Although orgasm is similar in men and women there are important differences. The woman needs much more time for arousal in order to achieve orgasm, whereas the man is able to have his climax without entering into much foreplay. In the male, orgasm is accompanied by ejaculation of seminal fluid, and once ejaculation has occurred the penis soon loses its erect form and becomes limp, whereas women are capable of having multiple orgasms, perhaps two or three over a short space of time.

Although the actual process of orgasm is always the same, the experience and intensity vary considerably as do the mysteries and myths surrounding it. During the early months of sexual intercourse it is common that orgasm is not reached and reaching a climax becomes more frequent as a relationship lengthens. Some women very seldom reach an orgasm and it is estimated that in the region of 10 per cent of women never do.

There are many reasons why women may not achieve an orgasm during sexual intercourse, though they may reach a climax by self-stimulation or masturbation: ignorance of the sexual act, embarrassment about her genital organs, failure of communication about which aspect of love-making pleases her, pretence of orgasm in order to satisfy the man and other emotional factors which time and patience often cure. Sometimes simple education in love-making, adopting different positions during intercourse, moistening the vagina with jelly if the natural secretions are not sufficient, produce immediate results, but in others the inability to achieve satisfactory orgasm can become a source of marital disharmony and expert help is needed. This can be obtained from a marriage guidance council and sex therapists. However unpalatable or embarrassing discussion on intimate sexual problems with a relative stranger may seem at first, expert help and therapy has helped many couples to overcome their sexual difficulties.

Finally, orgasm bears no relation to fertility, and failure to achieve an orgasm in no way influences conception or the ability to achieve a pregnancy.

Painful sexual intercourse

If love-making is difficult or causes pain, there is often a very simple explanation and medical advice should be sought if it persists. Pain during intercourse can occur either just at the entrance of the vagina or more deeply with the thrusting movements of the penis.

Pain occuring at the vaginal entrance can be due to a vaginal discharge or infection or it may be that the vagina is too dry and there is insufficient lubrication for the sexual act. This is common after the menopause when the vagina becomes more brittle.

Discharge or infection is treated with the appropriate drug and dryness is often helped by some lubricating jelly or hormone cream. In a woman who has not had intercourse the hymen will be unstretched and when intercourse takes place for the first few times there may be tenderness and some bleeding as the hymen is stretched and tears slightly. If difficulty continues the girl can be taught how to stretch her own vagina gently with the fingers or, rarely, a small surgical incision is necessary if the hymen is particularly tough.

Sometimes pain is caused merely because the muscles around the vagina go into spasm and tighten preventing penetration by the penis and there is often an underlying psychological cause for this: ignorance of the normal sexual act, fear of an unwanted pregnancy, guilt about sex drive are just some of the series of complex factors involved. It is easy to see how a vicious circle is set up as the woman gradually shrinks from the whole idea of intercourse which may become repellent as she associates the sexual act with pain rather than pleasure. Treatment is directed towards sympathetic understanding and instruction in sexual habits, and sometimes psychiatric help is needed.

Pain at the entrance to the vagina may occur after childbirth especially if a small cut has been made in the vaginal wall (episiotomy) which is commonly done to allow more room for the baby's head to pass through the stretched vagina. Sometimes this cut causes a scar which can be tender during intercourse or a little lump appears under the skin in the vagina where one of the knots has been tied. This can also occur following operations for prolapse. No treatment is usually needed and the symptoms resolve as the scar heals. Occasionally the vagina is narrowed slightly by the episiotomy or after surgical operations but it usually stretches satisfactorily with continued use. Surgery to widen the vaginal entrance or to refashion a scar may sometimes be indicated.

Deep pain during sexual intercourse may be due to abnormal positions of the womb and ovaries. If the uterus is retroverted (see Chapter 7) the penis may impinge on the uterus or ovaries causing a dull and sickening ache felt in the lower part of the abdomen. Other causes of deep pain are fibroids (see Chapter 4), infections of the womb and tubes (see Chapter 5), and endometriosis (see Chapter 4), and treatment of the underlying condition will improve things.

Masturbation

By this is meant the stimulation of the genitals in order to achieve orgasm with the hand or other objects. Usually masturbation implies the woman is stimulating herself but it also applies to stimulation of the genital organs by the male partner by means other than the penis. Traditionally thought to be unsocial and harmful, masturbation is a normal part of sexual development in both sexes. As girls and boys learn about their own bodies masturbation in the teens is commonly practised, and although its incidence diminishes with age and meaningful relationships many couples practise masturbation throughout life. Indeed, in some women it may be the only method of producing satisfactory orgasm. Contrary to the widely held beliefs often perpetuated by school and music-hall jokes that masturbation can cause deafness and blindness and all sorts of nonsensical illness, the only problem it creates is a feeling of guilt which is quite unjustified. However frequently practised masturbation causes no physical or mental harm whatsoever.

Homosexuality

The homosexual man or woman is attracted emotionally and physically to those of their own sex. Female homosexuals are known as lesbians, a word derived from the Greek Island of Lesbos which many thousands of years ago in Greek civilization was the home of a group of homosexual women. Though it is difficult to gauge the true incidence of adult lesbianism, it has been suggested that in the Western world 3 to 4 per cent of women prefer to share sexual and emotional interests with those of their own sex. There is, of course, the world of difference between a mature lesbian relationship and temporary homosexual tendencies that are so common in schoolgirls. The emotional attraction that a young girl may feel for a friend or an older woman or pop idol are perfectly normal feelings during the process of maturing and most girls will grow out of this phase.

Female homosexuality by no means necessarily implies physical contact, for lesbian relationships are very often deeply emotional and long-lasting. Though many lesbians prefer sexual relationships with each other many are heterosexual as well, though very often complete satisfaction and orgasm is only achieved with members of their own sex.

Many theories have been put forward as a cause of sexual homosexuality but few have been substantiated. It does appear, however, that it is unlikely that a homosexual will be born with that tendency and there is no scientific evidence to show that a female homosexual has more than her fair share of female hormones at birth or has any abnormality in the chromosome or make-up cells. It seems probable that a homosexual tendency is derived from home environment and parental attitudes. Some psychiatrists maintain that brutality at home causes rejection of one or other parent and a more masculine approach to life for the young girl. Others maintain that overprotection and smothering is equally as significant. What does seem clear is that a stable family relationship is important in preventing homosexual tendencies and the child brought up by one parent alone seems to be particularly vulnerable in this respect.

Female homosexuality is not an illness though even in modern society in many parts of the world it is still not accepted as normal. This fact coupled with the emotional instability that may occur from an insecure background can be a serious cause of mental anguish, and although many lesbians live a full, contented and happy life together it has been estimated that nearly a quarter undergo severe emotional stress needing the help of a psychiatrist.

Points to note

1 Sexual desire and satisfaction vary enormously with individuals and to some extent with times in life.
2 There is no 'normal' frequency for sexual intercourse. Some couples make love several times a week, others infrequently. 'Excessive' intercourse has no harmful effects.
3 It is not dangerous to have sex during a period or throughout pregnancy. Some doctors recommend avoidance of intercourse in the first few weeks of a pregnancy if any bleeding has occurred or if a previous pregnancy ended in a miscarriage.
4 Sexual intercourse after surgical operations is discussed in Chapter 14.
5 Spells of 'going off sex' are common in both sexes, often for no apparent reason. Sometimes the desire is reduced because

of fear of an unwanted pregnancy, guilt or just overwork and tiredness. Some drugs can lower sex desire, notably certain tranquillizers or even the contraceptive Pill. Being honest with your partner often improves things more than pointed rejection or excuses.

6 If you don't always get a climax during sex, don't think that you are unusual. Many women don't reach orgasm without finger stimulation first. Try a change of position with your partner underneath. This may stimulate the clitoris more readily especially if the vagina has been stretched by childbirth as the penis may not be gripped so well.

7 It is not essential to have an orgasm to get pregnant.

8 Masturbation causes no harm whatsoever.

9 If intercourse is painful and the vagina is dry, try smearing some vaseline or a jelly – called KY jelly and available at any chemist – inside the vagina. This helps to lubricate the canal and prevents friction. If difficulties arise for the first time after the menopause a visit to the doctor is often worthwhile. The usual cause is a brittle vagina due to lack of oestrogen and this can be considerably improved by hormone creams.

10 Sexual compatibility is not always immediate. It may take time and patience to achieve and inevitably has its ups and downs. As problems arise try and talk them over. Communication with your partner often does the trick. If you can't discuss things together or find you are getting nowhere, your doctor may help or refer you for specialist advice to a clinic dealing with sexual problems.

11 The infertile couple

About 10 per cent of married couples in this country are childless and formerly blame was attached usually to the female partner. It is now known that the male is at fault in about 35 per cent of cases of infertility, the female in another 35 per cent, and in 30 per cent there are factors present in both. Ninety per cent of married couples with no abnormalities should achieve a pregnancy within a year of trying and for this reason the word infertility is reserved for those who have failed to achieve a pregnancy by the end of this time. Unfortunately, despite considerable research into the causes of infertility, the success rate after treatment of either of the couple remains at the relatively low figures of 35 per cent. In order to understand why some couples fail to achieve a pregnancy it is important to consider some of the factors responsible in both sexes.

Pregnancy will result if the male produces spermatozoa of sufficient quantity and quality, and they are deposited in the vagina and move upwards through the neck of the womb via the body of the uterus to the fallopian tube. Although about 100 million sperm are produced with each ejaculation, by the time they have proceeded along the hazardous course from the vagina to the fallopian tube only a few hundred survive. Once in the fallopian tube they then have to swim for some way up the tube against the normal current. If the timing of arrival of a single sperm in the tube coincides precisely with the arrival of the egg from the female ovary which has been grasped by the tentacles of the tube and wafted down to meet the sperm, fertilization may occur. This timing is critical because the egg may only survive for thirty-six hours in the tube and the sperm one or two days.

Once conception has occurred the fertilized egg has to pass along the tube into the body of the uterus within three to four days; here it sinks into the already prepared lining of the uterus and hopefully it will then begin to grow and form an embryo.

Unfortunately, in about 20 per cent of pregnancies the developing embryo inside the uterus may be expelled and a miscarriage may result. With so many factors involved in producing the egg on the one hand and the male seed on the other, together with the perilous journey that both have to make before meeting, it is really quite surprising how often pregnancies do occur.

Causes of failure to conceive

Male factors

Perhaps no sperm or insufficient sperm are produced and there are many causes for this. The testicles may have been diseased in childhood or they may have been slow in descending at puberty; injury to the testicles, or exposure to large amounts of X-ray treatment, or certain drugs may lower the normal sperm count. It is well known that if the temperature in the sac containing the testes is much higher than normal the efficiency of the sperm diminishes. This may be due to varicose veins of the testicles or the wearing of athletic underwear which keep the scrotal sac at too high a temperature. Sometimes the passageway carrying the sperm may be blocked.

The testes may be able to produce sperm but ejaculation may not be satisfactory, may occur prematurely, or rarely the testes or penis may develop abnormally. Sperm may be correctly deposited in the vagina but may be unable to swim due to disease of the male prostate gland which affects their mobility.

Female factors

A single egg must be produced by the ovary some twelve to fourteen days before the next menstrual period. The fallopian tube must be healthy and normal so that the egg can be conveyed towards the uterus. The lining of the womb must be correctly prepared for receiving the fertilized egg so that implantation and further growth may occur. The neck of the womb must not act as a barrier to the passage of the sperm and should liberate clear colourless fluid at the time that the egg is released to attract the sperm to travel through into the womb and along to the tube. Simple lack of knowledge of the correct timing of intercourse, ignorance or fear of the sexual act, and a host of emotional factors may all play a part in delaying conception.

Investigation of the infertile couple

Just because a pregnancy has not been achieved after one year the couple should not take this to mean that they are infertile, and the initial consultation and examination by the doctor will often do much to remove these fears; it is surprising how often a pregnancy will result once reassurance has been given. Significant information may be gained from the questions asked at initial interview. In the man a history of injury or disease of the testicles, smoking and drinking habits, the use of particular drugs and the nature of ejaculation may give a clue to problems. Examination of the testicles may reveal discrepancy in size or some abnormality of the penis or varicose veins in the region of the scrotal sac.

In the female it is important to know whether the periods are regular and whether the menstrual flow each month is normal. If this is so ovulation is almost certainly occurring. Painful periods, though a nuisance, do usually indicate that ovulation is taking place. Some women can tell when ovulation occurs around the middle of the cycle because of abdominal discomfort midway between the periods accompanied by a little blood-stained jelly-like material from the cervix. If the periods are irregular,

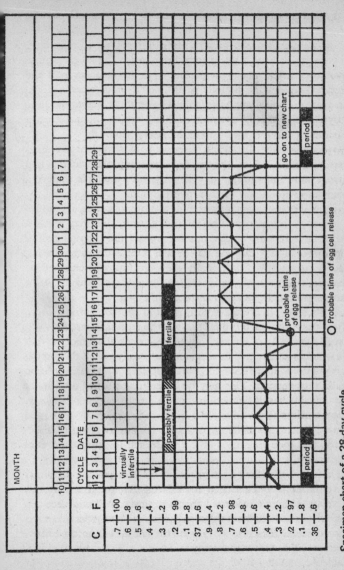

Specimen chart of a 28-day cycle
Time when conception is most likely. An example of temperature variation at different times of the month

○ Probable time of egg cell release

or the amount of menstrual flow is very scanty, ovulation may be deferred.

The frequency and timing of sexual intercourse is important. In order to achieve a pregnancy intercourse should take place two weeks before the next period, and this is so even if the interval between the periods is not exactly four weeks. If the periods come every six or seven weeks or three weeks, the time of ovulation is usually constant and still occurs about twelve to fourteen days before the onset of the next period.

It is important that frank discussion of sexual habits takes place because it is a well-known fact that simple explanation and correction of misconceptions will often help a couple achieve a pregnancy without any further investigation.

General examination may exclude any obvious cause for failure to achieve a pregnancy. The internal examination may reveal a spasm or tightening of the muscles around the external genital organs which may indicate that sexual intercourse is not taking place satisfactorily. Occasionally the womb may be enlarged by small innocent muscle lumps called fibroids (see Chapter 4) or the ovaries may be enlarged and contain cysts.

A tilted or retroverted womb is often thought to be a cause of infertility though it is doubtful whether this is in fact relevant. Usually the body of the womb meets the neck at an angle so that the womb itself is tilted forward and can easily be felt by internal examination. Sometimes the womb is in a backward position called retroversion. This may be a perfectly normal occurrence and usually has little significance in preventing a pregnancy. Occasionally the womb is tilted backwards because it is dragged down by previous inflammation or a condition called endometriosis and then treatment of the cause will improve chances of conception.

Having established that there is no abnormality in either partner and having excluded any existing general disease process the couple can be reassured that a pregnancy should occur. If this fails to happen after eighteen months or two years or if there is a particular reason to investigate the couple earlier the following tests are usually undertaken.

Examination of the male sperm

This is usually done in one of two ways. A specimen of sperm is produced by masturbation and is examined within four hours in the pathological laboratory. Sexual intercourse should be avoided for forty-eight hours before producing a specimen, but if embarrassment precludes a masturbation sample, sperm may be collected following withdrawal during sexual intercourse immediately before orgasm.

An alternative satisfactory method of analysing sperm efficiency is to withdraw a fresh quantity of sperm from the vagina with a syringe within six hours of sexual intercourse (post-coital test). The specimen is then examined under a microscope, the number of active sperm is counted, and their behaviour noted. This test may show that the sperm are not able to swim through the cervix or are killed off in the vagina before reaching the cervix. The normal cervix produces a thin watery discharge at ovulation time which is particularly attractive to the sperm. If this fluid is too thick and not of the correct consistency the

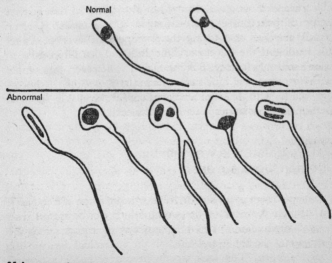

Normal

Abnormal

Male sperm types

sperm will not be able to enter the cervix. This occurs if there is any infection in the vagina or if the cervix itself is inflamed or eroded.

Tests to determine whether the egg is shed

Ovulation testing can be simply done by temperature record-ings. The woman takes her temperature with an ordinary thermometer every morning on waking and notes the tempera-ture change that occurs. The temperature in the first twelve to fourteen days of the menstrual cycle should be fairly constant but as ovulation occurs there is a dip followed by a rise and the temperature remains elevated throughout the second half of the cycle until the period comes again when the temperature will drop to its normal level. This temperature change occurs because ovulation causes the hormone progesterone to be liberated by the ovary which raises the body temperature.

It is best to continue temperature recordings daily over three consecutive cycles so that a pattern emerges which not only shows whether ovulation occurs but also when, so that correct timing of intercourse can be judged. Understandably, some women may feel that taking their temperature every morning only highlights the emotional difficulties and that intercourse to order is not satisfactory. For the majority, however, this simple procedure may give much information and specimen tempera-ture charts with relevant explanations are available in most doctors' surgeries or outpatient departments.

Tests to determine whether the fallopian tubes are open

Two methods are used, both involving the injection of a coloured dye through the neck of the womb which can be traced with X-rays (salpingogram) or by laparoscopy as it passes into the womb along the tubes and out into the abdominal cavity if the tubes are open. The laparoscopy procedure needs a general

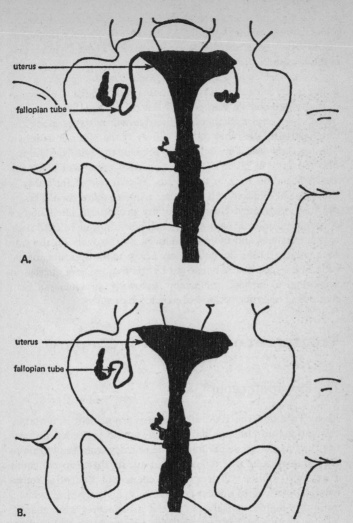

uterus

fallopian tube

uterus

fallopian tube

A.

B.

The injection of dye to show up abnormalities:
A. shows the tubes normal; B. reveals a blockage in
the fallopian tube on the right side

anaesthetic and therefore admission to hospital for a day is necessary. A salpingogram (X-ray) can be done without an anaesthetic and is usually quite tolerable. There is some discomfort similar to the insertion of an intra-uterine contraceptive device. The choice of procedure will depend on the policy of the particular hospital and its gynaecologist.

If the dye can be seen to spill out of the ends of the tubes, no blockage exists. Sometimes the dye will not pass along the inner parts of the tubes or will collect at the outer ends into a blind-ending sac. This will either prevent the egg from getting into the tube at all or if fertilization does occur will block the channel leading back to the uterus. If only *one* of the tubes is shown to be blocked and the other is open, there should be no bar to a pregnancy. Nor is there any decrease in likelihood of conception, because both ovaries will still continue to shed their eggs alternately and the egg produced by the ovary on the side of the blocked tube can find its way across to the opposite normal tube. This fact is well borne out by the frequency of success in achieving a normal pregnancy following previous surgical removal of one tube because of an ectopic pregnancy.

Treatment of the infertile couple

The low sperm count

An average of 60 to 100 million sperm are present in a normal ejaculation and although only a single sperm is needed to fertilize the female egg so perilous is the journey from the vagina to the fallopian tube where fertilization occurs that a sperm count of below 20 million will decrease the chances of conception somewhat, a count of 10 million considerably, and anything below 5 million is highly unlikely to succeed in achieving a pregnancy, though conception has occurred with a count as low as 1 million.

If a low count is found a second specimen is usually examined after the couple have abstained from intercourse for at least five days beforehand. If the second count remains low the testicles are examined to ensure that they are of normal size and consistency, and to exclude any visible abnormality such as varicose veins in the vas or fluid causing distension of the sac of the scrotum. Both these conditions are common causes of impaired sperm production and easily correctable by surgery. Sometimes there is an obstruction in the vas tube which can be diagnosed by injection of a contrast dye and taking X-rays. Again this blockage is readily amenable to surgical treatment with an often dramatic improvement in the sperm count.

If no abnormality of the testicles is detected blood tests can be done to detect whether the hormones responsible for producing sperm are insufficient and sometimes a small piece of testicular tissue is removed for microscopical examination. Injections of male hormone (testosterone) or pituitary hormone, produced by the part of the brain responsible for initiating sperm production, may improve a low sperm count but results are not always satisfactory. Further investigation and treatment is usually undertaken by a urologist. Artificial insemination with the husband's semen (AIH) may be worthwhile.

Complete absence of sperm

Orgasm and ejaculation may be occurring normally but when a specimen is tested no sperms at all are present on two successive occasions. Here there is either gross impairment of sperm production which may be due to a general disease process, injury to or abnormality of the testes that may have occurred in childhood, but often no cause is found on investigation. A specimen containing no sperms is unlikely to be improved by medication and the couple may be forced to consider AID (see later section) or adoption.

Failure to ovulate

Although temperature charts give a good clue as to whether ovulation occurs, if there is no satisfactory rise in temperature ovulation is probably not taking place and this must be confirmed by admission to hospital for a few days for blood and urine tests to confirm whether there is any fault with the hormones produced by the ovary and brain necessary to promote ovulation. It is usual that during the X-ray examination or laparoscopy a small piece of tissue is taken from inside the body of the womb and examined under the microscope to see if the lining of the womb has been readily prepared for receiving a fertilized egg. If this procedure is done just before a period the pathologist should be able to tell whether the lining of the womb is satisfactory or not, which will help to confirm whether ovulation has occurred in that cycle.

Several drugs are now available that are capable of stimulating ovulation and the overall success rate in producing egg release in women who were not previously ovulating is about 50 per cent. Of course this is only half the battle and although ovulation may be promoted by drug treatment conception still has to occur before a pregnancy results. The commonest drug in use is called Clomiphene or Clomid. This drug works by acting as a booster to the ovary that may not be good at making eggs properly and it also has some central action on the brain stimulating hormone production. Treatment usually consists of one tablet a day from the second day of the menstrual cycle for five consecutive days; and a course of three to four months is usually advised. Temperature charts will show whether this treatment has achieved the required result. If not, then the dose may be increased to two or perhaps three tablets and the same procedure adopted.

Clomiphene is a safe drug with few side effects. Like most fertility-producing drugs there is a slight but definite increase in the likelihood of a multiple pregnancy.

Hot flushes may be noticed and occasionally the ovaries grow and form fluid-filled sacs called cysts which rarely cause any problems.

If Clomiphene fails to produce ovulation a combination of hormones usually liberated by the pituitary gland can be given in the form of tablets or injections. Treatment with these hormones is complicated and painstaking for patient and doctor. Because the drugs are powerful and the body's response sensitive, multiple pregnancies may result, and to guard against this and also to achieve maximum success the precise dose must be calculated for each individual. This treatment involves close co-operation between patient and doctor, and because of the sensitivity maximum success is achieved in specialized centres that have the sophisticated monitoring equipment necessary for such assessment.

Recently, a new fertility drug has emerged which acts in a totally different way. It is called Bromocriptine and has been shown to be particularly successful in promoting ovulation in those women who do not shed an egg because of absent periods caused by a particular hormone imbalance which also causes milk secretion from the breasts. By a complicated mechanism Bromocriptine stops the production of milk and at the same time changes the hormone production so that menstruation and therefore ovulation can recur. Because this treatment is particularly safe, with very few side effects, it has also recently been used successfully in those who do menstruate and ovulate normally but somehow never manage to conceive a pregnancy.

Blockage of the fallopian tubes

Blockage of the fallopian tubes as a cause of infertility is unfortunately all too common. It has been estimated that 25 per cent of all cases of female infertility are due to fallopian tube occlusion. Damage to the tubes by infection and consequent blockage may occur after childbirth, after a pregnancy is terminated or as a result of venereal disease (Chapter 5), and because the canal of the tube which has to transport the egg is no wider than a straw previous inflammation may cause irreparable damage.

Can anything be done to unblock fallopian tubes ?
This will depend on how much of the tube is blocked, the actual site of blockage, whether the tube is damaged as well as blocked, and whether one or both tubes are affected. It would seem a relatively simple procedure to operate on the fallopian tubes, cut

out the area that is blocked if the blockage occurs at the free end, or to remove a portion of the tube if it is blocked at the uterine end and implant the remaining healthy part of the tube into another site in the uterus. Though the surgical technique of tubal reconstruction is not difficult the results of tubal surgery are disappointing. This is mainly because the tubes are so delicate that despite meticulous operative care a blockage may re-form again after surgery. Best results are achieved when the tubes are not actually blocked but merely kinked or twisted into an unusual position. The site of blockage or degree of damage to the tubes is usually assessed by laparoscopy (see Chapter 14) and before surgical reconstruction is attempted all other causes of failure to conceive are completely excluded. Ovulation is confirmed, the sperm is examined, any vaginal discharge is treated and a post-coital test should demonstrate an adequate number of active live sperms swimming in a clear pool of fluid.

Newer techniques of surgery for operations of the fallopian tube are under investigation and encouraging results have been achieved in some specialized centres by operating with a special microscope using extremely fine instruments.

What about tube transplants?
Attempts have been made to substitute diseased or blocked fallopian tubes with healthy tubes removed during sterilization procedures from another individual. In practice this method has not proved successful mainly because of rejection of tissue by the recipient and also because the fallopian tube is not merely a channel for transport of the fertilized egg but also has important functions – enabling the small embryo to grow before it passes into the lining of the womb. It has been suggested that a diseased fallopian tube could be entirely replaced by another tissue, say a vein, but this also has proved unsuccessful for similar reasons.

Artificial insemination

This involves the artificial transference of semen into the cervix. This can be done using the husband's semen, known an AIH, or sperm from an unknown donor, AID. AIH may be indicated when during normal sexual intercourse there is inability of the sperm to be deposited in the vagina because of an anatomical fault of the penis or if ejaculation occurs too early. If the semen count is low, and particularly if the fluid surrounding the neck of the womb does not allow penetration of the sperm because of hostility, direct injection of sperm through the cervix is also helpful.

There are two ways in which artificial insemination with husband's sperm can be done. Either a small quantity of sperm produced by masturbation is injected with a syringe into the cervix at the correct time of ovulation by the doctor, or the couple can be taught how to use a simple cap device which the woman inserts on to the neck of the womb and which is connected to a thin rubber tube through which the husband may inject a specimen of his own sperm with a syringe. The cap is inserted over the neck of the womb in much the same way as a diaphragm contraceptive, and remains in place surrounding the cervix overnight allowing the cervix to be bathed in a pool of sperm in the hope that at least a few sperm will penetrate into the uterus. Many couples prefer to use this method which is more psychologically satisfying than the rather anonymous method of injection of sperm by the doctor. The results with the 'cap method' are encouraging and the cap and tube are available at most clinics.

Artificial insemination with donor semen (AID) is indicated if the husband has no sperm at all or when he is known to be a carrier of certain hereditary disorders. The donor must be carefully chosen to match the partner in appearance and to be free of disease. Apart from the emotional, ethical and legal implications of AID the couple will have to decide whether they would prefer to rear the child of an unknown semen donor rather than adopting a child. The donor is completely unknown and he has no knowledge to whom his semen has been given. AID is not yet widespread in the NHS but the general practitioner may be able to suggest specialist advice.

Although 35 per cent of couples who consult their doctor for infertility will achieve a pregnancy there will remain many who do not. As a measure of the problem of infertility it is important to realize the difficulties involved in adopting a child. The agencies for adoption in this country are overwhelmed by requests and it is as well for the couple having decided on this course of action to consult their doctor soon, for the assessment of suitability for adoption is a lengthy process.

In the future

Perhaps the most remarkable recent advance is the 'test-tube baby story'. This is, of course, a misnomer because test-tubes are not actually used in order to grow the fertilized egg. The principle here is that an egg is removed from the ovary just before ovulation by laparoscopy and the egg is grown outside the woman's body in the laboratory. Male sperm is then added so that hopefully conception will occur. If conception occurs the fertilized egg is then replaced directly into the womb either by injecting through the neck of the womb from the vagina or via the abdomen with the torch or laparoscope. The theory is marvellously simple but the execution equally as difficult. Success in this country has already been achieved on a few occasions and the first baby born by this method was safely delivered by Caesarian section in 1978. In theory this success has opened up a new world for those women whose fallopian tubes are irreparably damaged and whose only hope of a pregnancy is by fertilization outside the body. It is early days yet to assess the significance of this magnificent achievement and much further research is being undertaken in this field.

Points to note

1 About 10 per cent of married couples in this country are childless, the fault being shared equally between both sexes.
2 If you have been trying to get pregnant for over a year without

success talk things over with your doctor. There is often a simple explanation and the interview and examination may be rewarding.

3 The best time to have intercourse is as near to ovulation as possible, i.e. 12 to 14 days before your next period.

4 Much can now be done to improve infertility. Drugs are available which promote ovulation, a low sperm count may be improved and surgery for blocked fallopian tubes can be successful.

5 Try not to get discouraged if investigations and treatment do not produce immediate results. Success often takes time and a lot of persistence and it is well known that anxiety and worry about failure to conceive only make matters worse.

12 The years of change

Of all species the only female to live beyond the potential for reproduction is the human. Her improved environmental conditions have resulted in an earlier start to the periods and a later end. In the present generation the periods usually finish at about the age of 50, which is four years later than the average age in the last century.

The word menopause is taken to mean the time when the periods stop and they may cease abruptly or they may occur at increasing intervals and become more scanty. One complete year's absence of periods in this age group is usually accepted as the true menopause. The menopause has long been accepted as a single event in the ageing process, merely representing the gradual cessation of the ovaries functioning properly leading to the absence of the sex hormone oestrogen. It used to be regarded as a relief from the burden of fertility but current views suggest that the hormone changes in the years following the menopause are more akin to a deficiency state producing some extreme changes in the body. Women, of course, differ in their attitudes to the menopause, as do doctors. Those who harbour an unwelcome view of periods doubtless welcome the advent of the change; others regard this loss of reproductive function as the depressing end of an era.

For a variable time before and after the periods stop certain changes take place as the result of a gradual withdrawal of the sex hormone from the ovary as the ovary starts to become less and less effective. In some women these changes go unnoticed, but many who have successfully coped with menstruation, contraception, family and a career are greatly incapacitated by the physical and emotional changes that follow the menopause. As the ovaries start to fail the output of oestrogen decreases and this may lead to a variety of symptoms, some occurring at an early stage and others some years after the periods have ceased.

The commonest complaint is the hot flush or sweat where sensations of heat suddenly envelop the face, neck and chest and the skin may show patchy red blotches. Sometimes drenching sweats occur, and particularly at night they may be followed by distressing chills. The attacks usually last from a few seconds to half an hour but may persist for an hour or even longer. They may occur only once or twice a day or sometimes as frequently as every hour. They are particularly disturbing at night, interfering with sleep, tend to be more severe in anxious women, and are intensified by excitement or stress.

Emotional disturbances commonly occur and these vary from episodes of anxiety, depression, palpitations, headaches, insomnia, fatigue and weakness. In some women these appear to be specifically related to lack of oestrogen and in others they may stem more from an exaggeration of her own emotional pattern.

Time and an ever-dwindling supply of oestrogen contribute to changes in the woman's outward appearance. The skin loses some of its elasticity and becomes dry. The hair may lose its lustre and gradually become thinner. The skin lining the vaginal entrance also becomes dry and brittle making the vagina more prone to inflammation and sometimes causing discharge and irritation. Because of these changes sexual intercourse may become painful leading to marital difficulties. Similar changes occur in the lining of the bladder causing occasional burning on passing urine and sometimes involuntary leaking of urine on exertion (stress incontinence – see Chapter 7). Oestrogen deficiency may also affect the internal pelvic organs, and the supporting structures of the uterus and bladder lose some of their tone and strength, encouraging dropping of the womb or prolapse.

Two very important late effects of lack of oestrogen concern the bones and arteries of the body. There is good evidence to suggest that the long bones of the body and spine soften as oestrogen is withdrawn, increasing the likelihood of fractures, particularly at the wrist and thigh. Slight curvature of the spine is a normal consequence of ageing but this is increased if the bones become thinner in the post-menopausal years producing backache and joint pains.

It is well known that the incidence of coronary heart disease is much greater in men than women under the age of forty because oestrogen produced by the normally functioning ovaries protects against the laying down of cholesterol and other fatty substances in the arteries which tend to harden their lining. After the menopause, as the oestrogen hormone is withdrawn and its protective influence declines, the incidence of coronary heart disease in women approaches that of men.

It is important to realize that these effects of lack of oestrogen vary enormously in different women and in 20 per cent the cessation of menstruation may be the only apparent sign of having been through the menopause.

Treatment for those with menopausal problems

The major question is to what extent these symptoms are due to lack of oestrogen and therefore how much they can be prevented by replacement of the lost hormone. Investigations of these complaints by smear and blood tests may give helpful information as to the amount of oestrogens still naturally present in the body, but the results are often misleading.

There are those who believe that these changes should be regarded as a normal part of a woman's life and that the symptoms should be endured perhaps with the help of sedatives. A more considered view is that the complex changes are a deficiency disorder which should be corrected by the appropriate replacement therapy with the hormone that is lacking.

There is absolutely no dispute that treatment with oestrogens is extremely effective in curing hot sweats and flushes, and the dryness and discomfort in the vagina. Much more controversial is the beneficial effect that oestrogen may have on the psychological and emotional symptoms associated with the menopause and the extent to which oestrogen treatment for a prolonged time may prevent some of the degenerative disorders that occur in the bone and blood vessels. Women themselves have been largely responsible for stimulating interest in the problems and benefits associated with oestrogen replacement therapy, and although many questions remain unanswered it seems that a new mantle of respectability has begun to replace many old-fashioned concepts. Many family doctors will prescribe oestrogens for menopausal symptoms, others prefer treatment to be undertaken by gynaecological departments of a hospital. Recently, specialist 'menopause clinics' have been set up in various hospitals staffed by personnel specializing in counselling and treatment for women with problems related to the menopause and those merely seeking information about hormone replacement.

Which type of oestrogen is best?

As oestrogen replacement therapy becomes more popular so the available pharmaceutical preparations increase. Some of these are *synthetic*, in other words the oestrogen is made up, and some contain *natural* oestrogens, derived from animal and plant sources, which seem to be preferable. Some of the possible harmful effects of oestrogen therapy which will be discussed shortly can be prevented by using a tablet of oestrogen together with progesterone, rather similar to the Pill but in a very much lower concentration. Most preparations that are available, either oestrogen alone or oestrogen with progesterone, come in memopacks of twenty-one tablets and are taken in three-weekly cycles and most will produce a small withdrawal bleed or period in the week off treatment. Though this may be irksome to the woman who has finished her periods there seems to be a certain advantage in shedding the lining of the womb at monthly intervals as this helps in preventing a build-up of the hormone in the body. Some doctors prefer to administer oestrogen in the form of a small pellet placed under the skin and the effect lasts about six months. This method of administration has the supposed advantage that a tiny amount of hormone is liberated daily at a constant rate; because no tablets are necessary the woman is not continually reminded of her condition, and the minor side effects such as nausea and indigestion are usually eliminated. This is also the method of choice for women who have had a hysterectomy.

Oestrogen creams and pessaries can be very helpful as an addition, particularly for the dry and brittle vagina causing painful intercourse. Birth control Pills can occasionally be used in controlling menopausal symptoms when there is still a possibility of pregnancy but because these are synthetic preparations that contain relatively high doses of hormone, for the older woman who needs to supplement her waning oestrogen to control distressing symptoms small doses of oestrogen from natural sources are far superior and safer than any birth control Pill.

How long can treatment be continued?

This is one of the most controversial issues and not all doctors are in agreement. Many women find that as well as helping distressing symptoms oestrogen treatment makes them feel fit and well and look better and they may want to continue treatment in the knowledge that oestrogens afford some protection against bone thinning and fractures. With modern safer preparations of oestrogen and progesterone and regular supervision many doctors are happier to allow their patients to continue on oestrogens for a number of years though much has yet to be learnt about the long-term effects of treatment.

What are the disadvantages of oestrogen treatment?

Many women encounter minor side effects during the first few weeks of treatment with oestrogens, such as breast tenderness and swelling, nausea, fluid retention with increase of weight, and vaginal discharge. These usually settle within the first month or two of treatment. Weight increase can become a problem because any hormone containing oestrogen does increase tissue fluid and encourage appetite. Care must be taken not to overeat and to keep to small regular meals, especially in the woman who is overweight and has a tendency to obesity.

Bleeding from the vagina is not a serious complication but troublesome to the patient and must be reported to the doctor. If oestrogen treatment is started some months or years after the periods have stopped, *irregular* bleeding or spotting of blood can occasionally occur from the womb in response to this drug. How-ever, the physician has no means of knowing whether this is in fact the cause or whether there is a polyp or small growth in the womb that has incidentally caused bleeding. The only way to be sure is for the woman to have a D & C (see Chapter 14) and this will usually be recommended. In the majority of cases the womb is found to be empty and then the bleeding may be assumed to be due to oestrogens. Providing the tablets are taken as directed this bleeding usually ceases and may not recur. If bleeding occurs at the end of a three-week cycle of pills, whether of oestrogen or oestrogen with progesterone, this can be regarded as normal. Although the doses of oestrogen in the tablet are fairly standard, if the bleeding continues advice from the doctor must be sought.

Oestrogens can cause a rise in blood pressure which is usually temporary, the blood pressure returning to normal once treat-ment is discontinued. Most doctors will hesitate to prescribe oestrogens to women who have a natural tendency to raised blood pressure.

Perhaps the two most important anxieties of oestrogen therapy concern *blood clotting* and the possible association with *cancer*. It is well known that some oestrogens, notably the synthetic ones, change the character of the blood as it flows through the veins and may increase the likelihood of stagnation and possible thrombosis. For this reason, any woman with a history of pre-vious blood clotting problems or thrombosis is usually denied oestrogen therapy. However, most of the so-called natural oestrogens seem to have less effect on blood coagulation and the incidence of problems with these hormones is minimal.

For a number of years controversy has raged concerning the possible association between oestrogens and cancer of the breast and uterus. Like the contraceptive Pill which also contains oestrogen and progesterone, though in much higher doses, oestrogens given to post-menopausal women occasionally cause a feeling of lumpiness in the breasts and innocent breast cysts can occur. Breast swellings which persist should always be reported to the doctor. Certain cancers of the breast are known to be sensitive to oestrogen; that is not to say that they are caused by the hormone but a pre-existing growth may be accelerated by oestrogens. There is no direct evidence to suggest that oestrogen causes breast cancer though it is not given to a woman who already has the condition.

With regard to cancer of the womb, the position is not quite so clear cut. Although there is no direct evidence to link oestrogens and cancer of the lining of the womb it has long been known that giving oestrogens to women past the menopause gradually causes the womb lining to grow and thicken which may give rise to bleeding. Some authorities believe that this thickening is really a very early stage of cancer formation; others dispute this strongly. The possible association between cancer of the womb and oestrogens has stimulated much research all over the world and from the evidence put to the first International Congress on the Menopause in 1976 the Chairman summed up as follows: 'The recent study alleging an increased risk of cancer of the lining of the womb in women under oestrogen therapy is open to serious criticism. The consensus of participants appear to support the view that there is *no* direct cause or relationship between cancer of the body of the womb in women and oestrogen treatment but there is an urgent need for continued research in this field.'

It appears that when progesterone is given with oestrogen this affords protection to the lining of the womb and prevents overgrowth and therefore this method of administration has become popular. Some experts believe if women are to remain on oestrogen for some time the lining of the womb should be explored by D & C at yearly intervals in order to note any possible change in the microscopical appearance.

At the present time a nationwide survey in the UK is being carried out to collect information about patients receiving oestrogen replacement to assess the long-term effects. For now it seems that the safest method of treatment is a pure oestrogen given together with a progesterone for three weeks out of every four which will cause a small period at the end of each treatment cycle. Oestrogen treatment in women who have had a hysterectomy is much simpler and it is safe then to take a daily tablet of oestrogen without fear of bleeding or a six-monthly injection in the pellet form if the doctor suggests that treatment is indicated.

The success of replacement therapy depends on a good understanding between the woman and her doctor and the safety enhanced by regular check-ups during treatment.

Points to note

1 The menopause is the time when your periods stop and marks the end of your reproductive ability.
2 The age at which the menopause occurs varies, the average being between 45 and 50, and your periods may stop quite suddenly or become irregular and gradually fizzle out over a number of months.
3 For a certain time before and after your periods finally stop certain changes take place in your body as a result of the gradual withdrawal of oestrogen from the waning ovaries.
4 For many women these changes go unnoticed; others may complain of a variety of symptoms – the commonest being hot flushes, perspiration, mood changes, depression and dryness of the vagina causing painful intercourse.
5 Oestrogens given by tablet or in the form of pellets placed under the skin provide effective treatment.
6 Oestrogens may also be effective in preventing some degenerative conditions such as bone thinning, leading to fractures of the bones, and may induce a general feeling of well-being.
7 Suggestions that oestrogens cause cancer of the breast and uterus have not been confirmed. If pure oestrogens are given with progesterone in a combined tablet the risks are minimized.
8 Not all doctors agree about the value of oestrogen treatment. Your family doctor is usually in the best position to give advice. Help may also be obtained from menopause clinics attached to the gynaecological department of some hospitals where specialist counselling and advice is available.

13 Cancer of the breast and reproductive organs

Cancer is one of several conditions that occurs because the cells of the body multiply in a disordered way. The body is continually making new cells to promote growth and repair dead tissue. Normally these cells divide many millions of times in a perfectly ordered manner and the cells which belong to the particular part of the body will only function with their parent tissue. In cancer this division of cells is totally haphazard and jumbled up so that an abnormal area of growth arises. If all the cells are packed tightly together in one area a lump will be formed and this is why cancer may appear so often in this way. The word cancer is very emotive and often taken to be synonymous with incurable disease, but this is not necessarily so at all. Many cancers in the body are now curable and although the precise cause of the condition is still not known great strides have been made in medicine with its prevention and cure.

Cancer of the breast

Diagnosis

Breast cancer is the commonest cancer in women and about 20,000 new cases are diagnosed per year in England and Wales. The disease accounts for 11,000 deaths annually. Although no women is immune from breast cancer it seems to be less common in women who have their first child under the age of 25 and who breast feed their children. This does not of course mean that breast feeding protects against breast cancer, merely that the incidence of the disease is slightly less common in women who do breast feed. Many theories have been put forward to try and predict those women who are at special risk of getting breast cancer. For instance the susceptibility to breast cancer seems to run in families, and daughters of breast cancer victims are said to run twice the risk of contracting the disease themselves. The professional classes tend to develop breast cancer slightly more often than the lower social classes and it has also been suggested that women who menstruate for many years are more at risk than those who start their periods late and finish early.

A lump in the breast that is painless, does not become more prominent before periods, and does not disappear afterwards must be reported to the doctor. Though most breast lumps are not cancer the earlier the diagnosis can be made the better the chances of permanent cure. Recent change in the appearance of the nipple or a blood-stained discharge should also be reported straightaway.

If a lump is confirmed the family doctor may either give reassurance that it is harmless or will ask for specialist assistance to confirm whether the nature of the lump needs further investigation. If the specialist believes the lump to be innocent, aspiration by a needle may confirm the presence of fluid and the patient may be reassured that the swelling is an innocent cyst. If there is any doubt as to whether a swelling exists, or to its nature, a special screening test called mammography may help to make a diagnosis. Commonly, if a swelling is confirmed it is surgically removed because the ultimate exclusion of a cancer can only be made by the pathologist in the laboratory.

Treatment

Once a diagnosis of breast cancer has been established treatment is either surgical or by deep X-ray or hormone treatment, or a combination of all three. In selecting the correct treatment the specialist will consider the age of the patient, the particular type of cancer, the presence or absence of any spread of the disease beyond the breast, and any other factors that may influence the outcome of treatment in any particular individual.

If surgery is advised the choice lies between removal of the breast lump itself, removal of the whole breast, or the infinitely more extensive procedure of removing the breast together with part of the underlying muscles and also some of the lymph glands – tiny channels which drain the breast tissue and along which minute cancer cells can spread. These channels drain from the breast towards the armpits and therefore surgery will need to involve the removal of some of the muscle underneath the breast together with these lymph glands. Because this procedure is more radical than merely removing the lump or the breast itself, it may produce discomfort after surgery because the arm on the affected side is liable to be painful and swollen for some time. Like so many treatments in medicine, controversy over which surgical procedure is best for any individual still continues. Although the larger operation is still performed in certain cases many surgeons now prefer the more minor forms of operation, perhaps accompanied by radiotherapy treatment.

Deep X-ray treatment and hormone therapy are usually given in addition to rather than instead of surgery. There are special circumstances where these treatments are indicated alone.

Can breast cancer be prevented?

The answer to that question is no, but the condition may certainly be diagnosed at an extremely early stage by self-examination of the breasts and a yearly visit to the doctor (see Chapter 3).

Cancer of the cervix

Diagnosis

The womb consists of two parts: the entrance or neck (cervix), and the body, which acts as a bed for the developing embryo in pregnancy. The neck and the body are made of very different tissue, the neck being firm and fibrous and the body soft and muscular. For this and other reasons cancer of the neck of the womb behaves in a different way from the body, in respect of speed of growth and ability to spread; therefore the treatment and the ultimate prognosis differ as well.

Cancer of the cervix is the commoner of the two and can occur at any age but the incidence is highest in women between forty-five and fifty. This type of cancer causes about 2,000 deaths each year in England and Wales and is responsible for 4 per cent of all deaths from cancer in women. The symptoms to look out for are irregular bleeding not associated with periods, bleeding after sexual intercourse, or bleeding after the periods have ceased at the menopause. Sometimes instead of bleeding there is a foul-smelling vaginal discharge.

There are harmless causes for these symptoms (see Chapter 2) but a visit to the doctor is indicated if irregular bleeding or a discharge persist, particularly in those over forty. The doctor will normally examine the internal genital organs with a torch and if the cervix looks in any way suspicious referral to the gynaecologist for further investigation is usual. The specialist may advise admission to hospital for two or three nights so that a sample of tissue can be removed from the suspicious area of the neck of the womb (biopsy – see Chapter 14) and sent to the pathology laboratory for microscopic examination. Though the treatment of cancer of the cervix becomes more difficult once the disease has been present for some time, thanks to a very simple test that can be performed by any doctor, cancer of the cervix may be suspected at a very early stage before any visible changes can be seen or any complaints exist.

This test is known as the *smear* test; sometimes called a 'pap' test after Dr Papanicolaou, an American physician who first discovered that scrapings from the neck of the womb examined on a glass slide could detect very early cancer cells. Dr Papanicolaou's findings formed the basis for the cervical smear test that is now carried out by family doctors, family planning clinics and gynaecologists.

How is the smear test done?

The cervix is first exposed by the doctor inserting a small spreading instrument into the vagina. The external surface of the cervix is lightly scraped with a wooden spoon and the invisible scrapings transferred to a microscope slide which is sent to the laboratory for examination. The whole procedure should be painless and takes a few seconds to perform. The smear test is not usually done during a period or if there is any bleeding as the presence of blood will make interpretation difficult.

The normal surface cells of the cervix appear in a certain pattern. This pattern can change into an abnormal arrangement under certain circumstances which can only be detected by a microscope with a magnification many hundred times greater than the naked eye could see. Hence the cervix may appear healthy to the doctor when the scraping is taken but laboratory examination may show an abnormality.

What is an abnormal smear?

An abnormal pattern or arrangement of the surface cells of the cervix does not imply that a cancer exists. It suggests that further examination of the cervix is indicated because the cervix may be at risk of developing a cancer at some time in the future (pre-cancer). Because an abnormal smear may be caused by infection of the cervix or an erosion it is usual for the test to be repeated after treatment before any further action is taken. Pathologists classify the abnormal smear into three or four types according to the degree of change in the cells. If the repeat smear shows marked abnormal changes referral to the gynaecologist is usual.

How early should the first smear be done?

Medical opinion varies considerably; some suggest that the first smear test should be taken once intercourse is occurring regularly however young the girl may be as there is evidence to suggest that the incidence of cancer of the cervix in later life is related to frequent intercourse occurring in youth.

How often?

Again there are no hard and fast rules but most doctors agree that smears should be done every three to five years until the age of forty and yearly thereafter.

Is the smear test necessary after the menopause?

Yes – changes may occur on the cervix at any age, though if previous smears have been normal it is unusual for the pattern to change later in life as it generally takes years for a pre-cancer to develop into cancer proper. The main advantage of a yearly smear test in the later age group is that the doctor may examine the other genital organs at the same time.

With such a simple, quick, painless screening test available to all women it should be theoretically possible to eliminate cancer of the cervix but overall figures in England and Wales for the last ten years have not shown the expected diminution of women presenting with this disease – despite 2.5 million smears being done per year, at a cost of about £10 million.

There is good evidence from British Columbia in Canada and from the Grampian Region of Scotland where intensive screening programmes are widely advertised, encouraging all women to attend doctors or clinics at regular intervals for cervical smears, that the number of *new* patients attending with established cancer of the cervix has been reduced; but in most parts of the world there is only the poorest evidence that screening programmes make much difference. There are other problems as well: not every pathologist will interpret the smear pattern in the same way. False positive results may be seen if there is an infected cervix or a vaginal discharge, and this is one of the reasons why women are asked to re-attend six months after the last smear because of a 'doubtful' result. Very early cancer cells or changes on the cervix that predict a cancer may be difficult to see and the diagnosis is by no means always simple or clear cut. Furthermore, the finding of a positive or abnormal smear does not indicate cancer; the smear that shows abnormal cells merely gives a warning that a cervix which may be healthy at the time the smear is taken may after many years develop into cancer proper.

Ultimately a decision will have to be taken by the politicians and administrators in the National Health Service as to whether a national screening programme of enormous proportions can be afforded with the limited financial resources available for health care, so that all women can be encouraged to have smear tests.

Treatment: the positive smear (pre-cancer)

If on routine examination a cervical smear test shows the presence of abnormal cells then the smear is usually repeated after a short interval. If the second test confirms the findings further investigation is necessary. Either the patient is admitted to hospital and under anaesthetic a section of the neck of the womb is removed for pathological examination (biopsy), or the cervix may be examined in the outpatients by a very powerful microscope called a colposcope which enables the specialist to look at many layers of cells on the surface of the cervix to differentiate between a cervix which is merely very inflamed and one that has an early malignant condition.

If the microscopical findings indicate a cancer proper, however early it may be, then the treatment will consist of radiotherapy or surgery as discussed in the next section.

If the microscope examination shows that there is no active cancer but the appearance suggests that the cervix is at risk of developing a cancer in years to come (pre-cancer) then provided the whole of the abnormal area has been removed at biopsy and the patient wants to have more children, no further active treatment is undertaken, but reviews are frequently made of the appearances of the cervix by repeated cervical smears. Some gynaecologists will suggest that hysterectomy or removal of the whole womb should be considered as an alternative procedure in a woman past child-bearing years, purely as a preventative measure.

Cancer proper

If a definitive diagnosis of cancer is made by the pathologist after examination of the biopsy specimen in the laboratory, the treatment rests between removal of the womb (hysterectomy) and radiotherapy. In this country radium treatment is generally preferred for a cancer of the cervix, though some surgeons like to combine this with removal of the womb. Radium treatment is normally preferred to surgery because although surgical removal of the womb and the cervix seems to be a logical treatment the surgeon cannot always be sure that very minute particles of cancer remain in the lymph channels or elsewhere whereas radium treatment is usually effective in burning away the original cancer and any invisible deposits that may have spread beyond the neck of the womb.

Radium treatment (radiotherapy)

Actively dividing cancer cells are particularly susceptible to destruction by radiotherapy and this treatment can be given either externally, with a special machine that points rays at the particular cancer, or internally, when a small block of radium is inserted into the vaginal passage and destroys the cancer cells by direct application. Not every hospital in the country owns these very expensive radiotherapy machines and some women need referral to a local radiotherapy centre. Treatment often takes a few weeks because it has to be given slowly and intermittently for fear of damaging normal tissue. Most women tolerate this treatment well though it is common in the first few weeks to notice some nausea and tiredness. Bowel upsets in the form of diarrhoea are also common.

Cancer of the body of the womb

Diagnosis

This condition is less common than cancer of the cervix and usually occurs in older women between the ages of fifty and sixty. Because the cancer starts growing inside the body of the womb rather than on the surface there is no similar test to the cervical smear that can detect or predict the growth at a very early stage. Fortunately, though, the body of the womb is very sensitive to any foreign growth within its walls and will react by bleeding. Like the cervix, therefore, any irregular bleeding occurring between periods, and especially after the periods have stopped around the age of forty-five to fifty, must be taken seriously. The bleeding is usually painless and may be merely a pink or yellow discharge. Doctors usually regard bleeding that occurs six months after the periods have stopped as significant.

The first investigation that is usually done is a minor surgical procedure called a D & C. It merely consists of gently stretching the neck of the womb so that a fine spoon or scraper can be introduced through the neck into the body and any abnormal tissue can be removed and sent to the pathology laboratory for microscopic examination. Though irregular bleeding or bleeding that occurs for the first time six months after the menopause must be reported to the doctor, so that a cancer can be excluded, 90 per cent of women with these complaints are subsequently shown to have no significant abnormality.

Treatment
Luckily a cancer inside the body of the womb grows very slowly and because the womb has very thick walls, spread of the cancer beyond the womb is unusual and treatment in the majority of cases is entirely curative. Whereas cancer of the neck of the womb is normally treated by radium with or without surgery, removal of the womb and ovaries (hysterectomy) is the treatment of choice when the cancer is confined to the body. Some gynaecologists though prefer to use radium treatment before or after surgery.

Cancer of the ovaries

Diagnosis
Cancer of the ovaries accounts for about 5 per cent of cancers in women and 10 per cent of cancers of the genital organs. The commonest age of diagnosis is around forty, but the condition may arise at any time. Early diagnosis is unfortunately not easy because the ovaries are situated inside the abdomen and there is no direct access to them from the outside. Many ovarian cancers are unsuspected and are only found during a routine internal examination by the doctor when the ovary may be felt to be swollen.

This emphasizes again the need for frequent examinations and is one of the reasons why an internal examination is always performed at family planning clinics, well-women clinics, and cervical smear clinics, in the perfectly fit woman without any gynaecological symptoms.

Some cancers of the ovary liberate a lot of fluid and this may cause swelling and discomfort in the abdomen, often accompanied by a feeling of acidity in the mouth or heartburn. A visit to the gynaecologist is often worthwhile if 'middle-aged spread' occurs suddenly.

Treatment

If internal examination reveals an ovary that is larger than it should be, surgery is usually advised so that a piece of ovary can be removed for microscopical examination. Sometimes the surgeon will be able to diagnose a cancer on naked eye examination during surgery and further treatment will then depend on the age of the patient and whether the growth is confined to the single ovary or has spread to involve the other ovary or other tissues in the body.

The usual treatment in the forty-year-old woman is to remove the ovaries and womb, because although the opposite ovary may appear normal there may be a very early spread of cancer cells which can only be detected by the pathologist and the cancer can also spread to the womb. External radium may sometimes be suggested after surgery.

Of all cancers of the genital system the ovary is the most responsive to certain anti-cancer drugs. Recent research has indicated that certain very powerful drugs are able to stop the abnormal growth of cancer cells in certain types of ovarian malignancy and it is common practice to suggest treatment with one of these drugs following surgery in order to rid the body of any remaining cancer cells and to prevent a recurrence. Some of these treatments are a little unpleasant and may cause nausea and a general feeling of ill-health as the drugs are powerful and tend to affect normal as well as abnormal tissues. Frequent supervision of drug treatment including blood tests is undertaken by the doctor.

Cancer of the external genital organs (vulva)

Diagnosis

Cancer of the vulva is rare and occurs usually in the over-sixty age group. An ulcer or a warty lump on the vulva that may discharge or bleed is usually noticed first. Sometimes intense irritation around the vagina may precede the occurrence of a lump and this symptom should be reported to the doctor. The finding of small tender nodules in the groin may be significant. Unfortunately, many women who have noticed some abnormality of the external genital organs for the first time in their sixties may be too embarrassed to consult their doctor until the ulcer has grown and has caused recurrent discharge or bleeding which becomes a nuisance, by which time curative treatment is difficult.

Treatment

Surgery rather than radium treatment or drugs is the treatment of choice. Because spread from a cancer of the vulva on one side occurs early and tends to involve the opposite lip and some of the lymph channels draining into the groin, curative surgery is an extensive procedure involving removal of the vulval area and some of the glands in the groin. As with most cancers the outcome will depend largely on the stage the disease has reached by the time a diagnosis is made, and although a lump appearing on the lip even at a late age does not necessarily signify cancer, early consultation with the doctor is essential so that if need be a small piece may be examined for microscopical examination.

Points to note

1 Although most breast lumps are not cancerous let your doctor have a look if you come across a swelling that persists or gets bigger.
2 Examination of your own breasts at regular intervals between periods is worthwhile.
3 If you notice any change in the appearance of the nipple or get any discharge from the breasts inform your doctor.
4 Breast screening with special instruments (mammography) may detect a swelling before it can be felt or seen.
5 Regular cervical smears may prevent an unsuspected cancer of the cervix from occurring later in life.
6 Don't ignore irregular bleeding that occurs between periods, after intercourse or after the menopause. There is probably a simple explanation but it is better to be safe.
7 Remember – the earlier a cancer is diagnosed the greater the chance of a complete cure.

14 Surgery

Going into hospital

Going into hospital can be a worrying time. Apart from any individual anxieties about your own treatment, complicated arrangements at work or home involving other people may be necessary during your stay in hospital and perhaps when you get home. Although it may be impossible to give accurate information, your doctor should be able to give you a rough idea of how long you will be in hospital, what you will feel like after surgery and what sort of thing you will and will not be able to do on return. Convalescence can usually be arranged after major surgery and the medical social worker should be able to help with this and other social problems. There is usually one attached to your ward and the sister in charge can arrange a meeting.

Those responsible for planning your admission to hospital for surgery will have noted the time of your periods as most surgeons prefer not to operate during a period. If your period starts a day or two before you are due to be admitted, let the hospital know as the operation may have to be deferred.

Most hospitals like patients to be admitted twenty-four or forty-eight hours before surgery because blood tests and investigations may need to be carried out while you are in the ward and the anaesthetist will want to check that you are fit for surgery. If you have been unwell recently or have a bad cold, particularly with a raised temperature, the doctors may postpone your operation until you are fully recovered. If you suffer from any allergies or know you cannot tolerate certain drugs because of previous bad reactions, let the doctors know.

One hour or so before surgery an injection called 'premed' (short for premedication) is usually given into your thigh or arm muscle. This usually makes you feel drowsy, dries the mouth and relaxes the body, generally helping the anaesthetic to work better.

Some people are particularly frightened by the idea of being put to sleep or anaesthetized with a mask over the face. This method is not generally used and it is normal for an anaesthetic to be given by an injection.

The pubic hair is generally shaved completely before major surgery whether it is to be performed through an opening in the abdomen or from the vagina, to prevent contamination of the operating area. Surgeons' attitudes to shaving before minor surgery (D & C, laparoscopy, cauterization to cervix) differ. Some consider that shaving is unnecessary, and others prefer to clip or shorten pubic hair.

Aperients or suppositories are usually given the night before to ensure the bowels are empty.

Once round from the anaesthetic the woman may be aware of a tube leading from a vein in the arm to a bottle containing either a colourless fluid (sugar) or blood, called a drip. This is common practice for major operations because surgery is a stressful event for the body and fluid is lost during anaesthesia causing some dryness. For the first twenty-four hours after surgery, oral intake of fluid and food is restricted so as not to cause any nausea or sickness and the fluid in the drip merely acts as food which can be absorbed through the vein and into the body. The drip is normally removed twenty-four or forty-eight hours after surgery by which time drinking is encouraged and a light diet started.

By the second or third day the scar is beginning to become less painful but cramp-like wind pains can occur as the bowel is starting to work again. A general anaesthetic tends to cause a temporary paralysis of the bowel and it takes a few days for the bowel to re-establish its normal motion. The first sign of bowel activity is the passage of wind from the top or lower end usually followed by a bowel action by the third or fourth day. If the bowels have not opened by this time an aperient is usually given or suppositories are inserted into the back passage.

By the fifth or sixth day the skin of the incision has healed together completely and the stitches or clips are removed. All surgeons have their preference for closing the skin of a scar; some use small staples or clips, others use silk stitches that have to be removed, and others use dissolvable sutures. Removal of clips or stitches is a procedure that many dread, but most women are equally surprised to note how painless it really is.

Activity is encouraged in order to restore the blood circulation and even if enforced bed-rest is necessary it is important to move the legs and ankles to prevent the blood from stagnating. Discharge from hospital is usual between ten and fourteen days after surgery.

These remarks are intended as guidelines only, as post-operative recovery and healing vary for each individual, with the type of operation, and particular hospital ward routine.

Operations through the vagina

D & C (scraping of the womb)

This minor surgical procedure is the commonest operation in gynaecological practice and is as valuable to the gynaecologist as a chest X-ray is to the physician. D & C stands for Dilatation and Curettage and involves the passing of a sharp-ended spoon-

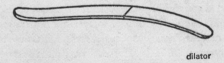

dilator

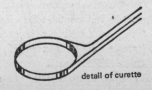

detail of curette

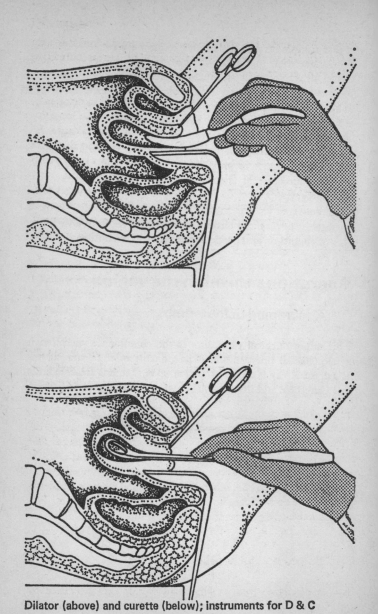

Dilator (above) and curette (below); instruments for D & C

shaped instrument through the neck of the womb into the body so that the lining of the body can be gently scraped (curettage) and the tissue obtained can be sent to the pathologist for examination. In order to be able to pass the instrument into the uterus the cervix has to be stretched by a series of metal instruments, each slightly larger than the previous one (dilatation). Generally the amount of stretching that is needed is minimal because the curette is thin and in women who have had babies and therefore have a naturally wider external opening to the neck of the womb the scraper can be used without any stretching beforehand.

Because the lining of the womb undergoes many changes with different gynaecological conditions, microscopical examination by the pathologist will give a clue as to the causes of certain complaints such as menstrual disorders, abnormal bleeding, infertility and the exclusion of cancer.

Sometimes the D & C can be therapeutic as well as diagnostic. For example, following a miscarriage bleeding may occasionally persist and a D & C is necessary to ensure that the contents of the womb are completely emptied. A D & C performed for heavy periods can sometimes reduce the menstrual flow for several months or years.

The whole procedure takes only a few minutes and is usually performed under general anaesthetic. Some hospitals prefer an overnight stay after an anaesthetic and some favour the procedure done as a day case. Under certain circumstances the D & C can be done without an anaesthetic, especially if only a minute specimen is required for diagnostic purposes. This usually involves the use of a suction apparatus attached to a special fine curette. There is a little discomfort during the procedure, which takes a few seconds only, comparable to that experienced during the insertion of an IUD. There may be a small amount of bleeding for a day or two afterwards but there should be no pain. The next period usually comes at the expected time.

Operations on the cervix

Vaginal discharge due to a cervical erosion can be cured by applying a heated wire to the outside of the cervix, destroying the surface cells and allowing new skin to cover the cervix (cautery).

This is usually done under general anaesthetic, but minor forms of erosion can be treated by touching the cervix with an acid stick in the outpatients or by freezing the cervix with a special instrument. Again this procedure is quite painless but the discharge may well increase for a while and occasionally this may last for a few weeks. The doctor may want to examine the cervix after six weeks to ensure the surface has healed and new cells have grown over completely. It is best to avoid sexual intercourse or the use of internal tampons for a few days after cauterization.

Cervical biopsy

The word biopsy means the removal of a small piece of tissue, which is then suitably prepared in the laboratory so that microscopical examination may be done. A general anaesthetic is usually necessary depending on the size of tissue that needs to be removed. Sometimes a large piece of tissue has to be examined, for example if there is an abnormal cervical smear test or if there is a suspicious-looking area on the cervix. This procedure is called a cone biopsy because a wedge of tissue is removed in the shape of a cone.

Small biopsies can be taken in the outpatients but usually admission to hospital for twenty-four to forty-eight hours is advised. If larger biopsies are necessary such as the cone, hospital stay may be extended for a few days.

Cervical stitch for recurring miscarriage

Some women tend to miscarry pregnancies in the fourth or fifth month due to cervical incompetence (see Chapter 9) and require a stitch inserted around the neck of the womb in order to prevent the cervix from opening. This is done under general anaesthetic at twelve to fourteen weeks of a subsequent pregnancy, necessitating a hospital stay of two to three days. The stitch remains in place during the pregnancy and is usually removed at thirty-

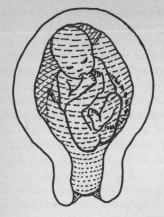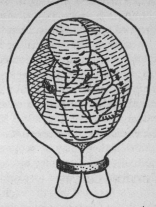

A. Bulging membrane in dilated canal   **B.** Encircling stitch tied about the cervix

Cervical stitch to prevent miscarriage

eight or thirty-nine weeks simply by cutting the knot. Success rates in maintaining the baby inside the uterus are high.

Repair of a dropped womb (prolapse)

In Chapter 7 it was seen that when the womb drops it drags with it the bladder in front and the rectum or back passage behind because these structures are initmately connected to each other. The principle of surgery involves the replacement of the dropped parts back into their original position together with tightening the muscles that surround the lower end of the vagina to ensure that the dropping does not recur.

If the neck of the womb itself has dropped very low it is sometimes removed. Some surgeons prefer to remove the whole of the womb (vaginal hysterectomy) together with tightening the stretched muscles to prevent any possibility of a recurrence of the prolapse and to eliminate any potential problems that may develop in the womb in later years. There are no hard and fast rules as to whether the womb is repaired or removed and each gynaecologist will have his own preference, and will take into account the degree of prolapse, the age of the patient, and any coexisting gynaecological conditions.

Recovery from vaginal operations is usually quick. Because there is no scar in the abdomen there is little pain and full mobility is possible within twenty-four to forty-eight hours. It is common practice for a tube (catheter) to be inserted into the bladder after surgery so that urine can drain freely and this catheter is usually removed after forty-eight hours or five days depending on the preference of the surgeon. When the tube is removed there may be some difficulty in starting to pass water normally and there may be some stinging while the bladder and the urethra get used to working again. Sometimes a wedge of gauze is inserted into the vagina at operation to prevent bleeding and this is usually removed with the catheter.

The average stay in hospital after major vaginal surgery is between ten and fourteen days. On discharge from hospital and over the first week or two it is quite common to notice some brown staining from the vagina or slight red loss. If bleeding persists or increases in amount the doctor should be consulted. Small strands of stitches may be passed from the vagina as they dissolve in the first week or so and this has no significance. Other general aspects of after-care will be considered in the section on hysterectomy (see later this chapter).

Operations through the abdomen

Laparoscopy

First introduced into this country fifteen to twenty years ago, laparoscopy is now one of the commonest gynaecological operations, and represents a major advance in diagnosis and treatment. The word laparoscopy simply means 'looking into the abdomen' and the instrument, which is really a modified torch, is called a laparoscope.

The main advantage of the instrument depends on the fact

that the entire contents of the abdomen can be examined through a tiny cut just below the navel without the need of a full scar so that discharge from hospital is normal after twenty-four hours compared with the usual post-operative in-patient stay that a formal operation requires.

The common uses for laparoscopy include testing the fallopian tubes for infertility (see Chapter 11), female sterilization (see Chapter 8) and for the diagnosis of unexplained pain thought to be gynaecological in origin.

Though it is possible to perform laparoscopy under local anaesthetic the majority of surgeons prefer full anaesthesia. A needle is inserted just below the navel into the abdominal cavity through which gas is passed so that the abdomen is blown up to a volume of approximately two litres. The gas ensures that vital structures such as the bowel float upwards leaving a clear space for the torch to be inserted. When the abdomen is blown up sufficiently a sharp hollow instrument is passed through the same cut under the navel and the torch inserted through this so that a view of the womb, ovaries and tubes is obtained. Sometimes a separate little cut is made in the lower part of the abdomen through which another instrument can be passed to pick up various structures and bring them into view.

For female sterilization the fallopian tubes are grasped in turn through an instrument passed down the laparoscope and an electric current is transmitted via the instrument so that a part of the tube can be burnt and destroyed (cauterized).

Instead of burning sections of the tubes, with the laparoscope a ring or clip can be positioned on a segment of the tube, effectively blocking the channel through which the fertilized egg passes – each surgeon will have his own preferential method.

No special after-care is needed. There may be one stitch in the navel, which either dissolves or needs to be removed within a week. Some discomfort and swelling in the abdomen may be experienced and it is not uncommon for pain under both shoulder blades to be noticed for a few hours, due to some gas still remaining in the abdomen. Discharge from hospital is usual within twenty-four hours.

Laparotomy

This word is used to describe any surgical operation involving an incision or cut into the abdomen. Laparotomy is performed in order to make a diagnosis of abdominal pain of unknown origin, or to remove a swelling due to a cyst, or a fibroid.

Most gynaecologists place the cut across the lower abdomen, just above the pubic hair line so that when healed it is covered by the pants. This incision heals extremely well, gives good access to the surgeon, and is cosmetically satisfying. Sometimes the cut is made in the middle of the lower part of the abdomen running up and down between the navel and the pubic hair line. This approach is usually used if the surgeon is dealing with a very large swelling or if surgery is expected to be difficult, because this incision gives better access. If a scar is already present from previous surgery then the common practice is to go through the same scar rather than place a second incision in the abdomen.

Hysterectomy

Although many of the previous remarks apply equally to hysterectomy as other abdominal procedures, this operation is surrounded by so much mystique that it deserves special mention.

Hysterectomy is the surgical removal of the whole womb and is by far the commonest major gynaecological operation. Almost always the body and the cervix of the womb are removed together and this operation is called a 'total hysterectomy'. Very rarely the neck of the womb is left behind, when the operation is called a 'sub-total hysterectomy', but this operation has little place in gynaecological practice. Unfortunately, these words have become muddled and when women talk about partial and complete hysterectomy they may not be referring to removal of part of the whole womb but whether the ovaries have been removed as well. The Americans are fond of using the expression 'pan hysterectomy' to denote removal of the womb and the ovaries.

The fact is that hysterectomy implies removal of the womb

alone, and if the ovaries are conserved, as they generally are when the womb is removed for a benign condition before the menopause, there is no change in sexual feeling, femininity or ageing process because the womb is simply the baby bed and has no hormone function of its own. The ovaries, on the other hand, are the primary sex organs; they are responsible for producing the hormone oestrogen which is vital for so many feminine functions in the body (see Chapter 12).

If the uterus needs to be removed for a benign condition and the ovaries appear normal then most surgeons do not remove the ovaries provided that the woman is still menstruating. Once the menopause is reached and hysterectomy becomes necessary, there is a greater tendency for removal of the ovaries as a routine because they are now functionless, do not form oestrogen any more, and the likelihood of a cancer developing in the existing ovaries increases somewhat with age. The decision as to whether normal ovaries are removed or preserved in the younger woman is a balance between possible trouble in the remaining ovaries in later years and the effects of loss of oestrogen. If the ovaries are removed while the woman is still having periods and has not reached the menopause the sudden withdrawal of hormones can produce quite marked hot sweats and flushes after surgery but these can be controlled by replacement therapy with the oestrogen in the form of tablets or injections.

What are the reasons for having a hysterectomy?
Certain conditions demand removal of the womb but in others the decision is much less clear cut. Hysterectomy is generally advised if there is a local malignancy in the womb; if there are large fibroids, giving rise to symptoms; if there is a hormone abnormality leading to heavy menstruation which has not responded to conservative therapy: if the tubes or ovaries are severely diseased by inflammation or endometriosis. Other indications for hysterectomy such as sterilization or as a purely preventative measure against malignancy or severe pain with the periods are less well defined.

Before the advent of medical treatment with hormones and a better understanding of the causes of certain gynaecological problems, hysterectomy was the treatment of choice for the majority of conditions and certainly in the United States it is estimated that 25 per cent of all women aged fifty and over have had their womb removed and close to half a million hysterectomies are performed each year and increasingly in younger women. In Europe the emphasis on surgery is less and a more conservative policy is adopted where possible.

Abdominal or vaginal hysterectomy?
The uterus can be surgically removed through a cut in the abdomen (abdominal hysterectomy) or through the vaginal passage (vaginal hysterectomy); the latter operation is often referred to by patients as 'the suction method' though no suction is used. Abdominal hysterectomy is by far the commoner of the two operations as it is generally technically simpler, especially if the womb is enlarged, and permits a thorough inspection of the rest of the abdomen, at the same time.

As there is no scar in the abdomen when the uterus is removed through the vagina, pain after surgery is less and recovery may be quicker, but this method is generally reserved for the woman who has a uterus small enough to pass through the vaginal entrance, and is ideal if a degree of dropping, or prolapse, exists as well.

How long to recover?
Though recovery from hysterectomy is variable the normal inpatient stay is between ten to fourteen days. It is important to realize that the first week or two at home are really an extension of being in hospital.

A period of convalescence is invaluable in those who have a large family or little help at home. Tiredness and fatigue is very common for the first few weeks after surgery as a natural part of the healing process. Housework should be kept to a minimum, lifting heavy weights discouraged, but gentle exercise such as walking is beneficial. Some vaginal discharge or even slight bleeding with the passage of small pieces of stitch should not cause anxiety – this is quite normal. There may well be mild aches and pains in the lower part of the abdomen for the first few weeks as the muscles knit together. Provided the wound is well healed a daily bath is fine and there is no reason for a woman not to drive a car for short journeys within two weeks of discharge from hospital. No special diet is necessary but a good fluid intake is important, and overindulgence in food is not advised.

The follow-up visit is usually five or six weeks following surgery. The doctor will examine the scar and the vagina to ensure that internal healing is satisfactory. If there is a vaginal discharge or slight bleeding by the time of this check-up it is due to some scar tissue or healing matter situated at the top of the vagina where the neck of the womb was removed; this is easily treated either by applying an acid stick in the outpatients, or by cauterization with a hot wire. It usually takes about three months for complete recovery from hysterectomy but this is enormously variable. Some women are able to return to light work within two months of surgery, and others may take up to six months before they feel fit enough to resume their normal activities.

What about sexual intercourse after hysterectomy?

Doctors usually recommend that intercourse be avoided for four to six weeks following hysterectomy, though this is only a rough guide. If hysterectomy is done through the vagina the inside of the vagina has a scar along its length and early intercourse may irritate the healing tissue. With abdominal hysterectomy there are no stitches in the vagina but there is a scar across the upper end of the vagina where the cervix previously was located. Thus the vagina ends in a blind tube and no communication exists between the vagina and the inside of the abdomen after hysterectomy.

Though early intercourse will cause no harm it is not unusual for slight bleeding or discharge to follow, caused by irritation of the healing scar. If this recurs the doctor should be consulted as sometimes the scar tissue needs to be touched with an acid stick or cauterized. Similarly, bleeding or discharge not necessarily provoked by intercourse may occur spontaneously several weeks after hysterectomy. This should not cause any alarm but again a visit to the doctor is indicated if bleeding per-

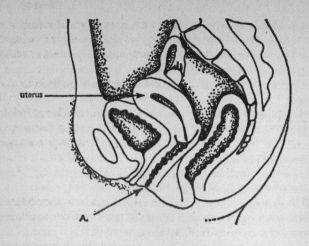

uterus

A.

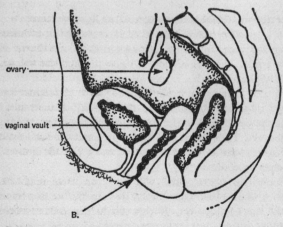

ovary

vaginal vault

B.

Before and after hysterectomy
(Note that the length of the vagina shown in A.
before hysterectomy is not shortened in B. after
hysterectomy)

sists. Contrary to popular belief there is no physicial reason why intercourse should cause pain or discomfort to either partner. Some authorities believe that removal of the cervix alters sexual satisfaction but this is seldom true.

The length of the vagina is slightly shortened particularly after vaginal hysterectomy but this is usually temporary as the walls of the vagina are very elastic and capable of stretching. Painful intercourse is much more likely to be due to lack of hormone if the ovaries have been removed, and treatment with oestrogen cream is helpful.

What else may be affected?

The space previously occupied by the uterus in the abdomen is immediately filled with loops of intestine and the position of the remaining abdominal organs is unaltered.

If the ovaries are retained ovulation and hormone production continues for a number of years. The mature egg which is about the size of a full stop simply gets absorbed in the body every month. Because ovulation occurs in a cyclical fashion many women may continue to get symptoms of abdominal swelling, breast tenderness and backache about the time the periods would have been due though no bleeding occurs. Treatment is the same before as after hysterectomy (see *Pre-menstrual tension*, Chapter 2).

There is no alteration in feminine attributes after hysterectomy, neither does abnormal hair growth occur. The female body always contains a small amount of male hormone which may cause some excess of facial hair as a normal result of advancing age. Hysterectomy with or without removal of the ovaries does not increase this tendency.

There is no reason why excessive increase in weight should occur. Obesity following surgery is usually due to overeating, though it is common for some weight to be put on as a result of inactivity during the convalescent period.

If the ovaries need to be removed in the woman who has not reached the menopause, hot sweats and nightly perspirations can be troublesome. Treatment with tablets or an implant of oestrogen is usually the cure (see Chapter 12), and the doctor may advise that replacement with hormones is continued for some time.

One of the most difficult features to assess is the psychological reaction to hysterectomy. To some women removal of the womb brings complete relief from unwelcome menstruation and pain. Others may feel that they have been finally deprived of their reproductive function and take time to get over this emotional loss. Mental depression occurring for the first time after hysterectomy is well recognized but not always easy to predict. It seems, however, that the well-motivated woman who understands the indications and implications of hysterectomy is unlikely to suffer psychologically.

Points to note

1 If you need to make domestic arrangements while you are in hospital, try to make sure that any help you have can be extended for a few days after you get home.
2 If your period is likely to coincide with admission to hospital or you happen to have a bad cold or feel unwell, let the hospital know in good time. It may save you an unnecessary visit as your operation may have to be deferred.
3 Don't forget to tell the doctor if you have any allergies or certain drugs do not suit you.
4 Your periods can return any time after surgery. There is no set pattern but the first period after minor surgery may be heavier than usual. Obviously you won't get any periods if you have had a hysterectomy.
5 Hysterectomy implies removal of the whole womb (body and neck) but not necessarily the ovaries.
6 The ovaries are generally conserved unless they are diseased or you are near or past the menopause, when they are inactive.
7 Hysterectomy does not cause loss of femininity, hair growth, premature ageing or an alteration in desire for sex.
8 Excessive weight gain after abdominal operations is usually due to overeating.

9 If it is necessary to remove both ovaries before your menopause, the hormone oestrogen that the ovaries make can be
   replaced by tablets or injections after surgery.

10 Removal of *one* ovary does not cause any change in the body.
   The remaining ovary takes over the function of two and provides all the oestrogen necessary.

Appendix

The gynaecological consultation and examination

The lengthy waiting period for an appointment, the uncertainty of a strange doctor in unfamiliar surroundings, and worry about an internal examination may cause many women attending a hospital outpatient department for the first time considerable anxiety. Inevitably, there needs to be a certain amount of routine in a department dealing with large numbers of patients every day and though it may seem that the various preliminary details before the consultation – such as history and personal details, the measurement of blood pressure, recording of weight – are performed with bewildering speed by different members of the clinic staff, these details give vital information to the doctor before the consultation.

While waiting to see the doctor it is helpful to try and marshal some thoughts about your complaint so that as clear an account as possible may be given. For example, if you have a pain in the abdomen the doctor will want to know:

When the pain started and what brought it on ?
Is it constant or does it come and go in waves ?
Is it severe or is it just a dull constant ache ?
What makes it better and what makes it worse ?
Does the intensity of the pain bear any relation to the periods ?

Consultation

The doctor will probably start by asking about your chief complaint, and this is often followed by a series of set questions; though at first sight some may seem to be irrelevant, the gynaecologist is trying to get an overall picture of how the particular problem is affecting you. There is certain information that the gynaecologist will always want to know:

What is the normal pattern of menstruation?
Has it altered?
When did the last period occur?
Was it normal?
Are there children from the marriage?
Were there any problems or complications with childbirth?
Does a discharge exist?
Is there any pain or difficulty with intercourse?
Is there a history of general illness or previous operations?

It is important that questions concerning contraception and sexual intercourse do not cause embarrassment as it is vital for the doctor to know if precautionary methods are used and what these are. For example the Pill or the intra-uterine device could be the sole cause of bleeding between the periods, or a vaginal discharge that has become heavy.

Examination

Again each specialist will have a routine for examination so that important signs of disease are not missed. This normally consists of a general examination, including feeling the breasts for any lumps and examination of the abdomen to exclude a swelling or areas of tenderness.

Internal examination is done either with the woman on her side or on her back. This is the most important part of the examination and it is useful if you can breathe gently and rhythmically during examination as this relaxes the muscles of the

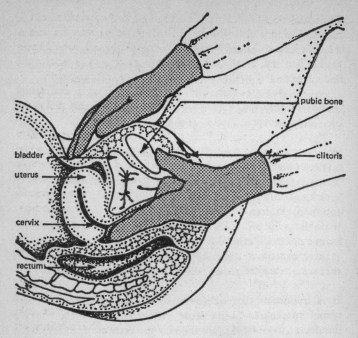

Examination of the pelvic organs with both hands

abdomen and makes it easier for the doctor to feel things. During
the internal examination a small metal torch is passed into the
vaginal passage so that the cervix can be seen. A cervical smear
is usually taken at the same time. The torch may feel a little
cold but apart from a slight stretching feeling there should be no
particular discomfort.

The second part of the examination involves feeling the internal organs with the fingers of one hand in the vaginal passage
and the other resting on the abdomen. As the doctor's fingers
inside the vagina press upwards the other hand on the abdomen
presses down, so that the womb can be felt between the two
hands and its size, position and consistency noted. It is necessary for the doctor to use both hands in this way because under
normal circumstances the uterus cannot be felt by merely feeling

the abdomen and therefore it has to be pushed upwards from the vagina. The specialist will then be able to tell whether the uterus is larger than it should be, perhaps due to fibroids (see Chapter 4) or softer than usual if a pregnancy is present. The ovaries are next examined by slight pressure on either side of the pelvis.

The whole procedure takes a few minutes only and many women are surprised and relieved to note how simple and painless the procedure is.

Those who have not had sexual intercourse will be particularly apprehensive about the first internal examination. They may be reassured that the doctor will be aware of this after the history has been taken and will use a very small torch which hardly stretches the vagina at all. If internal vaginal examination is impossible the doctor may insert a finger into the back passage, or occasionally will suggest that examination takes place under anaesthetic at a future date.

Internal examination may cause a little bleeding or discharge afterwards and this is quite normal.

Hospital referral to the gynaecologist does not necessarily imply disease. Often the family doctor is merely requesting a second opinion and in many instances reassurance can be given that there is no abnormality or if a cause for the complaints is found it can be cured by explanation and medication rather than surgery.

Index

Gordon Bourne
Pregnancy £2.75

Having a child can be one of the most exciting and fulfilling experiences in a woman's life, provided she has the confidence that comes from knowing exactly what pregnancy involves. This comprehensive guide is written by Dr Gordon Bourne, Consultant Obstetrician and Gynaecologist at one of London's leading teaching hospitals. It provides full information, guidance and reassurance on all aspects of pregnancy and childbirth. An indispensable aid to the expectant mother, it will also be of great interest to her husband and family.

Dr Barbara Evans
Life Change 80p

For every woman undergoing the change of life, Dr Evans, Managing Editor of *World Medicine*, explains what is happening to your body, your emotions and your relationships: how the menopause affects you; how to cope with it; how and when hormone treatment can help; sex and the menopause; the risks of cancer. This book brings knowledge, expertise and hope to those suffering the physical and psychological problems of the menopause.

edited by Sigmund Stephen Miller
Symptoms £2.50
– the complete home medical encyclopedia

The new medical encyclopedia – accurate, comprehensive, easy to use, sensible – enabling the reader to track down any symptom of ill health and identify, quickly and accurately, the causal disorder. *Symptoms* will tell you exactly what is wrong, and guide you in what action to take, whether a simple home remedy, or whether to seek advice from your doctor. Each section of the book is written by a specialist in one area of the body, and there is also a glossary of medical terms, comprehensive cross-indexes, and a guide to maintaining a high standard of general good health.

Selected Bestsellers

☐	**The Empty Hours**	Ed McBain	£1.25p
☐	**Shanghai**	William Marshall	£1.25p
☐	**Symptoms**	edited by	
		Sigmund Stephen Miller	£2.50p
☐	**Gone with the Wind**	Margaret Mitchell	£2.95p
☐	**Robert Morley's Book of**		
	Worries	Robert Morley	£1.50p
☐	**The Totem**	David Morrell	£1.25p
☐	**The Alternative**	edited by	
	Holiday Catalogue	Harriet Peacock	£1.95p
☐	**The Pan Book of Card**		
	Games	Hubert Phillips	£1.50p
☐	**The New Small Garden**	C. E. Lucas Phillips	£2.50p
☐	**Everything Your Doctor**		
	Would Tell You If He		
	Had the Time	Claire Rayner	£4.95p
☐	**A Town Like Alice**	Nevil Shute	£1.50p
☐	**Just Off for**		
	the Weekend	John Slater	£2.50p
☐	**The Deep Well at Noon**	Jessica Stirling	£1.75p
☐	**The Eighth Dwarf**	Ross Thomas	£1.25p
☐	**The Music Makers**	E. V. Thompson	£1.50p
☐	**The Third Wave**	Alvin Toffler	£1.95p
☐	**Auberon Waugh's**		
	Yearbook	Auberon Waugh	£1.95p
☐	**The Flier's Handbook**		£4.95p

All these books are available at your local bookshop or newsagent, or can be ordered direct from the publisher. Indicate the number of copies required and fill in the form below

Name_____
(block letters please)
Address_____

Send to Pan Books (CS Department), Cavaye Place, London SW10 9PG
Please enclose remittance to the value of the cover price plus :

25p for the first book plus 10p per copy for each additional book ordered
to a maximum charge of £1.05 to cover postage and packing
Applicable only in the UK

While every effort is made to keep prices low, it is sometimes
necessary to increase prices at short notice. Pan Books reserve
the right to show on covers and charge new retail prices which
may differ from those advertised in the text or elsewhere